Common Diseases and Cure

Published by :
Lotus Press Publishers & Distributors

Common Diseases and Cure

Dr. Rajeev Sharma
M.D., D.Lit.

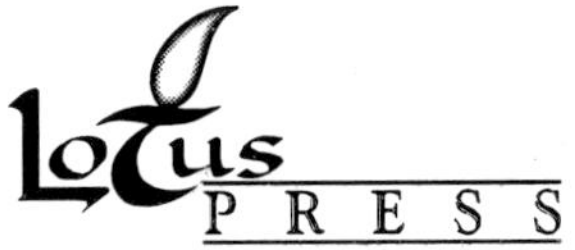

4735/22, Prakash Deep Building
Ansari Road, Darya Ganj,
New Delhi - 110002

Lotus Press : Publishers & Distributors
Unit No. 220, 2nd Floor, 4735/22, Prakash Deep Building,
Ansari Road, Darya Ganj, New Delhi- 110002
Ph.: 41325510, 9811838000
• E-mail : lotuspress1984@gmail.com
www.lotuspress.co.in

Common Diseases and Cure

ISBN: 81-8382-055-7

Attention Readers:

Every effort is made to ensures accuracy of material, but the publisher, printer and author will not be held responsible for any inadvertent error(s). In case of any dispute, all legal matters to be settled under Delhi Jurisdiction only.

Printed & Published by : **Lotus Press Publishers & Distributors,** New Delhi-02

Preface

'Common Diseases' and common man. Yes, this was the feeling in developing this book. From eye disorder to bladder infection all major ailments are included in this book, like asthma, constipation, arthritis, impotency, lencorrhoea, hair loss, acne, pimples etc. A separate chapter is included on today's largest nutritional disorder-obesity.

This book will help you in finding causes and appropriate treatment of your ailment. Though, you can not become a doctor, but you can understand your problem and know the treatment. In case you want to start your own prescription, on behalf of this book, you can start, but it is always advised to consult a proper physician first. The surgical aspect is only to be done by surgeons.

If you have any querry, you can write me with a reply envelop. If you want to consult me, first fix an appointment on phone and please don't come without appointment.

With thanks & regards—

Sincerely your's

Dr. Rajeev Sharma
Srijan—AAROGYA JYOTI®
Palm—11/03, Shipra Suncity,
Indirapuram, Ghaziabad (UP)
Ph.: 0120-3020206
E-mail: sharmarajeev100@rediffmail.com

A Brief About

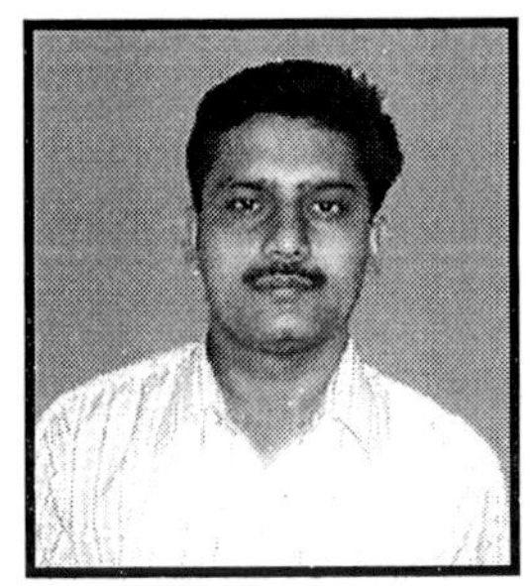

Dr. Rajeev Sharma

Dr. Rajeev Sharma is an eminent consultant of Homoeopathy, Yoga, Naturopathy and Alternative Medicine in India. He has written more than Two hundred books (200) in Hindi and English and around one thousand articles which have been published in various newspapers and magazines. He is also an Editional Board Member of the prestigious *Asian Homoeopathic Journal* besides many other newspapers and magazines.

Dr. Rajeev Sharma has written books on ayurveda, allopathy, homoeopathy, yoga, naturopahty, accupressure, magnetotherapy, reiki, water-therapy, massage and aromatherapy etc.

The books written by Dr. Rajeev Sharma are published by renowned publishers of India. Besides this he is doing editing and translation also. He is content provider to many magazines.

Dr. Rajeev Sharma has written books on all major ailments like diabetes, hypertension, obesity, stomach and respiratiory disorders, E.N.T. disorders, female disorders, UTI disorders, paediatric problems, head ache, stress and other mental problems and Sexual Disorders etc. You can fix an appointment for any of such problem.

Dr. Rajeev Sharma is Medical Advisor to Ralson Remedies (a homoeopathic manufacturer), and Dixit Pharmacy (Ayurvedic Manufacturer), Medical Examiner at the LIC and Medical Officer in U.P. Govt. He has received several prizes for his outstanding achievements. He has been awarded the *Best Author prize in Hindi* by the Ministry of Health and Family Welfare, Government of India and *Sarjana Puraskar by U.P. Hindi Sansthan,* Lucknow. He has delivered talks on All India Radio and lectures on Alternative Medicine in various Government and Non-government Organisations. He has written Advt. Scripts for the products of several companies.

He is working as Vastu Fengshui Consultant, Educational Consultant and Marriage and Behaviour Counsellor too.

He is delivering lectures and providing literature on Personality Development and Life Style Management also to the MNC's.

He has established an institute through which you can get certificates by correspondence in Accupressure, Massage, Yoga, Water Therapy, Diet Therapy, Naturopathy, Colour Therapy and Reiki besides other paramedical courses.

Dr. Rajeev Sharma is also a social activist. He has worked a lot against Addition and prevention of AIDS. Now a days, he is working to check the population growth of India with an NGO called 'Nav Chetna Manch'. He has worked for pollution control and human rights too and has received the World Human Rights Promotion Award. His name has been published in *LIMCA BOOK OF RECORDS* 2005. He has developed two websites too:-

www.newkamasutra.com: A site of love, romance and sex.

www.indiaalive.net: Patriotic site (Future planning)

Contents

1

Some Important Eye Disorders

CONJUNCTIVITIS

Conjunctivitis, also called pink eye, is a common condition in which the conjunctiva, the clear membrane covering the white of the eye and lining the eyelids, becomes inflamed.The affected eye becomes red and sore and may look alarming, but the condition is rarely serious. One or both of the eyes may be affected, and in some cases it begins in one eye then spreads to the other.

What Are the Causes?

Conjunctivitis may be caused by a bacterial or viral infection, or it may result from an allergic reaction or irritation of the conjunctiva for example, by smoke, pollution, or ultraviolet light.

Bacterial conjunctivitis, which is common, may be caused by any of several types of bacteria. Viral conjunctivitis can occur in epidemics caused by one of the viruses responsible for the common cold. It may also be due to the herpes simplex virus that causes cold sores. Conjunctivitis due to a bacterial or viral infection can be spread by hand-by-eye contact and is usually highly contagious.

Newborn babies sometimes develop conjunctivitis. This can happen if an infection is transmitted to the baby's eyes from the mother's vagina during the birth. This form of conjunctivitis is usually caused by the microorganisms responsible for certain sexually transmitted diseases, including chlamydial cervicitis, gonorrhea, and genital herpes.

Allergic conjunctivitis is a common feature of hay fever and of allergy to dust, pollen, and other airborne substances. The condition may also be triggered by chemicals found in eyedrops, cosmetics, or contact lens solutions. Allergic conjunctivitis often runs in families.

What Are the Symptoms?

The symptoms of conjunctivitis usually develop over a few hours and are often first experienced on waking. The symptoms generally include:

- Redness of the white of the eye.
- Gritty and uncomfortable sensation in the eye.
- Swelling and itching of the eyelids.
- Discharge that may be yellowish and thick or clear and watery.

The discharge may dry out during sleep and form crusts on the eyelashes and eyelid margins. As a result, the eyelids sometimes stick together on waking.

What Can I Do?

The symptoms of conjunctivitis can be relieved by bathing the eye with artificial tears. To avoid spreading infection, wash your hands after touching the eye and do not share towels or washcloths. Once the conjunctivitis has cleared up, vision is rarely affected.

If you are susceptible to allergic conjunctivitis, avoid exposure to triggering substances. Antiallergy eyedrops can be used to ease the symptoms. If an eye becomes painful and red, you should consult your doctor to rule out the possibility of a more serious condition.

What Might the Doctor Do?

Your doctor probably makes a diagnosis from your symptoms. If infection is suspected, he or she may take a sample of the discharge to identify the cause.

Bacterial conjunctivitis is treated by applying antibiotic drops or ointment. In such cases, the symptoms usually clear up within 48 hours. However, the treatment should be continued for 2-10 days, even if the symptoms improve, to ensure the eradication of infection. Viral conjunctivitis that occurs because of a herpes infection may be treated with eyedrops containing an antiviral drug. Although other types of viral conjunctivitis cannot be treated, their symptoms usually clear up within 2-3 weeks. Your doctor may prescribe eye-drops or oral antiallergy drugs if you have allergic conjunctivitis.

CORNEAL ULCER

An erosion in the cornea, the transparent outer part of the front of the eyes, is called a corneal ulcer. These ulcers can be very painful and, if they are left untreated, may cause scarring and lead to permanently impaired vision, blindness, or even loss of the eye. People who wear contact lenses are at increased risk of corneal ulcers.

What are the Causes?

Corneal ulcers may be caused by an eye injury, an infection, or a combination of both. A relatively small injury such as a corneal abrasion (left), can develop into a corneal ulcer if the damaged area becomes infected. A more severe injury, such as that caused by a caustic chemical, can produce an ulcer in the absence of infection. However, an ulcer that becomes infected may enlarge and penetrate more deeply into the cornea. Only rarely do infections cause corneal ulcers without prior injury. The most common of these infections are herpes zoster, known as shingles, and herpes simplex infections.

What are the Symptoms?

If you have a corneal ulcer, you may experience the following symptoms:

- Intense pain in the eye.
- Redness and discharge from the eye.
- Blurry vision.
- Increased sensitivity to light.

With an untreated infected ulcer, the infection may spread and permanently damage the vision in that eye and the eye itself. Consult your doctor immediately if you develop a painful, red eye along with blurry vision.

What Might Be Done?

Your doctor may place fluorescein eye-drops in the affected eye and examine it under blue light, using a slit lamp. He or she may also take a swab to identify the cause. If the dye reveals an ulcer, you may be given antibiotic or antiviral eye-drops to treat the infection. Even severe ulcers usually clear up within 1-2 weeks of treatment, but they can leave scars of treatment, but they can leave scars that permanently affect vision.

TRACHOMA

Trachoma is a serious, persistent eye infection that often causes permanent scarring of the cornea, the transparent front part of the eye. Although rare in developed countries, trachoma is one of the world's main causes of blindness. It affects about 400 million people, of whom about 6 million are blind.

Trachoma is due to the bacterium Chlamydia trachomatis, which is spread to the eyes by direct contact with contaminated hands or by flies. Trachoma is common in poor parts of the world, particularly in hot, dry countries that have poor sanitation and limited water supplies. Overcrowding encourages the spread of the trachoma infection.

To avoid becoming infected in a high-risk area, you should wash your hands and face regularly and avoid touching your eyes with dirty fingers.

What are the symptoms?

Initially, trachoma causes inflammation of the conjunctiva, the membrane that covers the white of the eye and lines the eyelids. Later symptoms include:

- Thick discharge from the affected eye that contains pus.
- Redness of the white of the eye.
- Gritty sensation in the eye.

Over time, repeated episodes of trachoma can cause scarring on the inside eyelids. The scars may pull the eyelids inward and cause the eyelashes to rub against the delicate cornea. Left untreated, the condition can lead to blindness.

What is the treatment?

In the early stages, trachoma is treated with antibiotic eyedrops or ointment. If the cornea has become scarred, sight may be restored by an operation called a corneal graft, in which a cornea from a donor is used to replace the scarred one.

CATARACT

If you have a cataract, the normally transparent lens of the eye is cloudy as a result of changes in protein fibers in the lens. The clouding affects the transmission and focusing of light entering the eye, reducing clarity of vision.

If cataracts are present from birth, total loss of vision may result. However, cataracts do not usually affect children or young adults. Most people over age 75 have some cataract formation, but visual loss is often minimal as only the outer edges of the lens are affected.

Cataracts usually develop in both eyes, but generally one eye is more severely affected. A cataract in the central part of the lens or one that affects the whole lens can cause total loss of clarity and detail in vision. However, the affected eye will still be able to detect light and shade.

What are the causes?

All cataracts occur as a result of structural changes to protein fibers within the lens. These changes cause part or all of the lens to become cloudy.

Changes in the protein fibers are a normal part of the aging process, but cataracts that develop earlier in life may occur because of an eye injury or from prolonged exposure to sun light. They may occur due to diabetes mellitus, uveitis, or long-term treatment with the chromosomal abnormality or Down syndrome.

What are the symptoms?

Cataracts usually develop over a period of months or years. In most cases, they are painless and usually cause only visual symptoms, such as:

- Blurry or distorted vision.
- Star-shaped scattering of light from bright lights, particularly at night.
- Altered color vision: objects appear reddish or yellow.
- Temporary improvement in near vision in people who were farsighted.

A severe cataract may make the pupil of the eye appear cloudy.

What might be done?

Your doctor may examine your eyes with a slit lamp and an ophthalmoscope. If your vision is affected significantly, he or she may recommend that the cataract is removed surgically and an artificial lens put in the eye. If there is no other reason for your visual deterioration, your sight should improve greatly after the operation. However, you may still need to wear glasses afterward.

GLAUCOMA

Fluid continually moves into and out of the eye to nourish its tissues and maintain its shape. In glaucoma, the flow of fluid out of the eye becomes blocked and pressure inside the eye rises. This high pressure may permanently damage nerve fibers in the light-sensitive retina and in the optic nerve, which carries nerve signals from the retina to the brain. Glaucoma becomes more common with age, and mainly affects people over 60 year of age. If untreated, the condition may cause blindness.

What are the types?

There are two common types and two rare types of glaucoma. Acute glaucoma develops suddenly, causing rapid loss of vision and severe eye pain. In contrast, chronic glaucma develops slowly and painlessly, often over many years. It may not cause noticeable symptoms until the eyes are badly damaged. Both types can run in families.

Secondary glaucoma occurs because of an underlying disorder, such as uveitis, or from using certain drugs such as corticosteroid eyedrops.

The other rare form, congenital glaucoma, is due to a defect in the drainage apparatus of the eye. Congenital glaucoma is present from birth and can lead to blindness. Secondary glaucoma can also result in blindness.

Glaucoma is diagnosed by measuring pressure in the eye using an instrument called a tonometer. Treatment should always be given urgently. Eyedrops are used first, to reduce pressure in the eye. In some cases, surgery is then necessary to increase drainage of fluid and prevent the build up of pressure in the eye. Correct treatment normally prevents further vision loss.

Retinal detachment

The light-sensitive retina of the eye is normally attached to the underlying tissue, but in retinal detachment part of the retina peels away from this tissue. The condition usually affects one eye only but without rapid treatment, can cause partial or total blindness.

Retinal detachment usually begins with a small tear in the retina. Fluid is then able to pass through the hole and separates the retina from the supporting tissues underneath. Tears may be caused by disorders such as severe near sightedness or eye injuries. In some people, tears appear as a result of scarring after a vitreous hemorrhage. Retinal detachment sometimes runs in families.

What are the symptoms?

Retinal detachment is painless, but its visual symptoms may include:

- Flashing lights in the cornea of the eye.
- Large numbers of dark spots in the field of vision.

If a large area of the retina has become detached, you may experience a cloudy ring or a black area across your field of vision. If you experience any of these symptoms, you should go to the emergency room of your local hospital or call your doctor immediately.

What might be done?

Retinal detachment is diagnosed by ophthalmoscopy, which is a technique used to examine the eye's internal structures. If only a small area of retina has detached, the tear may be sealed by laser treatment under local anesthesia. However, if a large area has detached, an operation under general anesthesia is necessary. If treated early, normal vision may be restored, but delayed treatment is less effective.

RETINOPATHY

Some long-standing diseases can damage small blood vessels throughout the body. If the blood vessels in the retina (the light-sensitive membrane at the back of the eye) are affected, the damage is known as retinopathy. Retinal damage varies according to the under lying disorder but can include leakage of blood from damaged vessels, loss of blood flow to some areas, and abnormal development of new blood vessels. Retinopathy may cause loss of vision.

One of the most common causes of retinopathy is diabetes mellitus. The condition can also occur as a result of high blood pressure, although vision is not usually affected in this case. Less frequently, retinopathy may be caused by AIDS, oxygen therapy in premature babies, or by sickle-cell anemia. Usually, only the underlying disease is treated. However, in diabetic retinopathy, laser surgery treatment of the retina itself can save vision.

EYE INJURIES

The eyelid-closing reflex and the bony socket around the eye help protect the eye from injury. However, eye injuries are still common, and in some cases blindness may result if the injuries are not treated promptly.

The most common injury to the eye is a scratch on the transparent cornea caused by a foreign body in the eye. Minor injuries of this type rarely damage vision permanently unless they develop an infection that remain untreated. However, penetrating injuries in which the eye is pierced by a tiny, fast-moving object, such as a metal chip from machinery, can lead to total loss of sight. Blunt injuries, such as those due to a blow from a fist or ball, may also endanger vision. Injuries can also occur by using caustic chemicals or by looking directly at the sun.

Most eye injuries can be prevented by the use of protective eyewear when working with dangerous machines or chemicals or when participating in athletic activities. Never look directly at the sun, even while wearing sunglasses.

what are the symptoms?

The symptoms of eye injuries differ according to the type and severity of damage, but symptoms may include:

- Pain and watering of the eye.
- Inability to open the eye.
- Bleeding under the front surface of the eye.
- Bruising and swelling of the skin around the eye.
- Reduced vision in the affected eye.

In the majority of minor eye injuries, first aid will often be helpful, but you should always seek medical attention for any eye injuries. If the injury was caused by a blow to the eye, involves a penetrating foreign body, or results in reduced vision, hold a clean, dry cloth over the injured eye and go to the nearest hospital emergency room.

What might be done?

Your doctor will probably assess the eye by ophthalmoscopy

and a slitlamp examination. Ultrasound scanning may also be used to look for a foreign body in the eye.

Most eye injuries only need treatment under local anesthesia, although some will require surgery under general anesthesia. Chemical injuries may be treated with corticosteroids.

Most eye injuries heal completely with prompt treatment. Sometimes corneal injuries leave a scar, and, if the lens is damaged, part of it may become cloudy. Sunlight may cause permanent damage to the retina, and separation of the retina from its underlying layer due to a heavy blow requires urgent treatment to prevent loss of sight. A serious eye injury can cause permanent blindness.

STYE

An infection at the root of an eyelash may result in the formation of a pusfilled swelling called a stye. Most styes are caused by Staphylococcus aureus, a bacterium found on the skin of many healthy people. Adults are less likely than children to develop styes, but, if you use eye makeup or wear contact lenses, you may be at increased risk.

A stye begins as a red lump on the edge of the eyelid. Over the next few days, the eyelid becomes swollen and tender, and a yellow spot may form at the center of the swelling.

What is the treatment?

Styes usually rupture, drain, and heal in a few days without treatment. You may be able to speed the process by placing a clean, warm, damp cloth on the stye for about 20 minutes four times a day. To avoid infecting other people or reinfection yourself, always wash your hands after touching the infected eyelid and avoid sharing or reusing personal items such as towels or washcloths.

If a stye does not heal in a few days or if the swelling becomes worse, see your doctor. He or she may prescribe a topical antibiotic, which should be put directly on the stye and the skin surrounding it.

However, if the stye persists, you may also need to take an oral antibiotic, after which the stye should clear up within 2-3 days. Styes are unlikely to cause long-term damage, but they tend to recur in some people who are prone to them.

CHALAZION

If an oil-secreting gland in the eyelid becomes blocked, the gland enlarges, creating a swelling called a chalazion. A chalazion may at first look like a stye, but unlike a stye it is not on the eyelid margin. Usually, the pain and redness associated with a chalazion disappear after a few days. However, if the swelling is large, it may cause long-them discomfort, and pressure on the front of the eye can interfere with vision.

What Might Be Done?

If your doctor diagnoses a chalazion, he or she will probably wait for several weeks before arranging any treatment because it will probably disappear on its own. Meanwhile, if the chalazion is painful or irritating, holding a clean, warm, damp cloth against it may help.

A persistent chalazion can be treated by simple operation in which a small cut is made in the inner surface of the eyelid and the contents of the swelling removed. The procedure is performed under local anesthesia and is painless.

PTOSIS

Drooping of the upper eyelid due to weakness of the muscle that raises it is called ptosis. The condition may be the result of a problem with the muscle or nerve that controls the eyelid. The sagging lid may partly or totally close the eye. One or both eye may be affected.

Ptosis is occasionally present from birth. If a baby's eyelid droops and it covers the pupil, his or her vision may not develop normally and early treatment is vital.

Ptosis in adults can occur as a part of the aging process, or it may be a symptom of myasthenia gravis, which causes progressive muscle weakness. If ptosis starts suddenly, it may be due to a brain tumor or a defective blood vessel in the brain. If you develop ptosis, see your doctor to rule out a serious underlying disorder.

What is the Treatment?

Ptosis in babies can be corrected by surgically tightening the eyelid muscle. If the treatment is carried out early, the child's vision should develop normally.

In adults, surgery for ptosis should be carried out only after any possible significant underlying disorders have been ruled out. Surgery is very effective for ptosis caused by the aging process.

WATERY EYE

Watery eye usually results from irritation of the eye by a foreign body such as a particle of dirt. Older people often have watery eye as a result of entropion, in which the eyelashes rub against the eye, or ectropion, in which tears do not drain away normally. The watering usually stops when the irritant is removed or the underlying condition is corrected. Watery eye may also occur as a result of a blocked nasolacrimal system (which drains tears), possibly caused by an infection of the eye or sinus infection.

Babies may have watery eyes because the nasolacrimal system is underdeveloped. Gently massaging between the corner of the eyelid and the nose may help. The condition usually corrects itself by age 6 months. Persistent blockage, at any age, must be treated by a doctor, who may clear the blockage by inserting a fine probe into the tear duct.

XEROPHTHALMIA

Xerophthalmia, which occurs mainly in developing countries, means dryness of the eye. The condition is caused by a dietary deficiency of vitamin A.

Left untreated, xerophthalmia leads to chronic infection and the cornea (the transparent part of the front of the eye) may soften and perforate. Infection may then spread inside the eye and blindness may result. Artificial tears may relieve dryness, but the main treatment is large doses of vitamin A.

2

Caries and Gingivitis

Caries

Medical term for tooth decay.Dental caries begin when bacteria in plaque eat away at the outer layer (enamel or cementum) of a tooth. Normally, these layers are strong enough to withstand invasion, but when the residue of built up food (plaque) remains on the teeth, it gives the bacteria a chance to work more steadily.

Tooth decay may start as a small spot on a tooth. Left untreated, it can destroy teeth, gums and even the bone around the teeth. The bacteria work their way into the tooth and into the pulp. The further the bacteria go, the more damage is done.

Early stage caries often go unnoticed. As the tooth deteriorates, it becomes increasingly sensitive to sweet, hot, or cold food. Removing the decayed area and filling the cavity is the usual form of treatment. For severe cases, removal of the tooth pulp (root canal treatment) or the tooth itself (dental extraction) is necessary.

People can prevent caries by reducing the amount of sugar and other refined carbohydrates in their diet. The next step is proper oral hygiene. The fluoride in toothpaste and flouridated water strengthens enamel.

Gingivits

Inflammation of the gums.Like the teeth, the gums (gingiva) are affected by plaque build up. Failure to brush and floss properly can result in an infection with bacteria that destroy the gums and the bones and teeth around them.

Most people pay insufficient attention to their gums and may be unaware of any trouble in this area until symptoms occur. In the early stages of gum disease (gingivitis), the gums bleed easily during toothbrushing. There may be pain and terndemess, the gums may be swollen, and there may be a discharge of pus, especially as the disease progresses.

Gingivitis can often be reversed simply through proper dental hygiene, including brushing regularly and flossing carefully. The use of either dental floss or interdental stimulators is essential in keeping the gums healthy and strong. Failure to take care of the teeth and gums can result in a worsening of the inflammation, to the point that the damage is no longer reversible and more extreme measures must be taken.. The gums can recede to the point that even healthy teeth can loosen and fall out.

3

Toothache and Erosion

Toothache

Pain in or around a tooth or teeth.

There are many causes for toothaches, but they all have one thing in common; they are the result of inflamation or injury to dental pulp. The most common cause of a toothache is simple tooth decay (caries) that irritates and can possibly affect the pulp of the teeth. As infection sets in, the pain increases.

The infection can progress to become an abscess. An abscess occurs when a pus-filled sac forms around the root. This can be painful and dangerous; the abscess infection can spread into the bloodstream. Interestingly, a burst abscess is often mistakenly thought to be a good sign, since it relieves the pain because there is no longer pressure.

Toothache always warrants the attention of a dentist. Sometimes the pain will go away for a while; this may be sign of a dead nerve, which needs to be addressed promptly if the tooth can be saved.

Erosion and Abrasion of Teeth

People who complain that their teeth are "wearing away" or becoming more sensitive to the cold aren't imagining things. But they may not realize that these symptoms are due to erosion and abrasion of the tooth surface that's almost entirely, if unintentionally, self-inflicted.

Dental erosion is a chemical process that gradually eats away at your teeth's tough outer enamel coating. Abrasion also removes tooth enamel, but by physical instead of chemical means.

Neither should be confused with cavities, or caries, which result from a bacterial process that can bore through not only the enamel but also the inner dentin layer of the tooth. Eroded or abraded teeth can change shape and colour as the yellowish dentin begins to show through the thinned enamel. More significantly, teeth can become ultra-sensitive to cold.

Erosion

The major culprit in erosion is acidity: the crystaline calcium salts that make up most of tooth enamel start dissolving below a pH level of 5.5. In most people the main offenders are the mild acids contained in many beverages and citrus fruits.

Surprisingly, according to a study on extracted teeth in the *General Dentistry*, the worst enamel erosion is produced by non cola drinks, such as ginger ale, Mountain Dew, Sprite, and bottled iced tea.

In this study brewed black tea, brewed black coffee, and root beer produced minimal erosion; colas were more erosive than these beverages but less so than the non cola drinks. There was no difference between the sugar-free and regular versions of these products.

Other sources of oral acidity include gastroesophageal acid reflux (GERD) and acidic medications, such as chewable vitamin C and aspirin tablets.

Saliva is an important defense against tooth enamel erosion. It dilutes and helps neutralize acids and contains minerals to replace those lost to erosion. Therefore, people who experience low saliva levels, or dry mouth, whether from disease, radiation treatment, or medication, have a higher risk of developing the problem.

Abrasion

It's ironic that the people most prone to abrasion are often the ones who are trying hardest to keep their teeth clean. Vigorous brushing with hardbristle brushes and abrasive pastes not only can wear away the tooth enamel but also cause the gum line to recede, exposing and removing the outer covering of the root and exposing the underlying soft dentin.

Worse, tooth erosion and abrasion can act synergistically. For instance, if you consume an acidic drink and brush immediately afterward, you can actually accelerate the erosive process by brushing away the softened outer surface. If you wait a bit, to give your saliva time to remineralize your teeth, you may not do as much damage.

Save your set of 32

The follwoing precausions will ensure that the minerals in your tooth enamel last as long as you do:

— Avoid acidic beverages when possible. If you prefer the aerated kind, drink it promptly, rather than sipping. Use a straw to help the acidic liquid bypass your teeth.

— Instead of brushing after drinking a high-acid beverage, thorughly rinse with water or use a fluoride rinse.

— Use only a soft-bristled regular or electric toothbrush. Brush with light pressure, using small, circular motions, rather than sawing away vigorously. Be especially gentle when brushing along your gum line.

— Don't have your teeth professionally cleaned more than two or three times a year. The polishes used at some dentists' offices can be extremely abrasive. So, too, some whiteners.

— If you suffer from dry mouth, stimulate your saliva flow by sucking on sugar-free hard candy, chewing gum containing the sweetener xylitol, or snacking on fibrous food such as carrots or celery.

— If you grind your teeth at night, ask your dentist about fitting a retainer like appliance that will protect your teeth.

— If erosion and abrasion have made your teeth sensitive to cold or other stimuli, switch to a desensitizing toothpaste. If your exposed roots have become extremely sensitive, ask your dentist about covering them up with a resin or composite.

4

Conducting Hearing Loss and Its Management

Any disease process which interferes with the conduction of sound to reach cochlea causes conductive hearing loss. The lesion may lie in the external ear and tympanic membrane, middle ear or ossicles up to stapediovestibular joint.

The characteristics of conductive hearing loss are:

1. Negative Rinne test, i.e. BC>AC.
2. Weber lateralised to poorer ear.
3. Normal absolute bone conduction.
4. Low frequencies affected more.
5. Audiometry shows bone conduction better than air conduction with air-bone gap. Greater the air-bone gap, more is the conductive loss.
6. Loss is not more than 60 dB.
7. Speech discrimination is good.

Management

Most cases of conductive hearing loss can be managed by medical or surgical means. Treatment of these conditions is discussed in respective sections. Briefly, it consists of:

1. **Removal of canal obstructions,** e.g. impacted wax, foreign body, osteoma or exostosis, keratotic mass, benign or malignant tumours, meatal atresia.

2. **Removal of fluid.** Myringotomy with or without grommet insertion.
3. **Removal of mass from middle ear.** Tympanotomy and removal of small middle ear tumours or cholesteatoma behind intact drum.
4. **Stapedectomy,** as in otosclerotic fixation of stapes footplate.
5. **Tympanoplasty.** Repair of perforation, ossicular chain or both.
6. **Hearing aid.** In cases, where surgery is not possible, refused or has failed.

Congenital causes of conductive hearing loss

- Meatal atresia
- Fixation of stapes footplate
- Fixation of malleus head
- Ossicular discontinuity
- Congenital cholesteatoma

Tympanoplasty

It is an operation to (i) eradicate disease in the middle ear and (ii) to reconstruct hearing mechanism. It may be combined with mastoidectomy if disease process so demands. Type of middle ear reconstruction depends on the damage present in the ear. The procedure may be limited only to repair of tympanic membrane **(myringoplasty),** or to reconstruction of ossicular chain **(ossiculoplasty),** or both **(tympanoplasty).** Recons-tructive surgery of the ear has been greatly facilitated by development of operating microscope, microsurgical instruments and biocompatible implant materials.

Acquired causes of conductive hearing loss

External ear Any obstruction in the ear canal, e.g. wax, foreign body, furuncle, acute inflammatory swelling, benign or malignant tumour or atresia of canal.

Middle ear (a) Perforation of tympanic membrane, traumatic or infective

(b) Fluid in the middle ear, e.g. acute otitis media, serous ofitis media or haemotympanum

(c) Mass in middle ear, e.g. benign or malignant tumour

(d) Disruption of ossicles, e.g. trauma to ossicular chain, chronic suppurative otitis media, cholesteatoma

(e) Fixation of ossicles, e.g. otosclerosis, tympanosclerosis, adhesive otitis media

(f) Eustachian tube blockage, e.g. retracted tympanic membrane, serous otitis media.

Myringoplasty

It is repair of tympanic membrane. Graft materials of choice are temporalis fascia or the perichondrium taken from the patient.

Ossicular reconstruction

It is required when there is destruction or fixation of ossicular chain. Most common defect is necrosis of the long process of incus, the malleus and the stapes being normal.

5

Acute Suppurative Otitis Media

It is an acute inflammation of middle ear by pyogenic organisms. Here, middle ear implies middle ear cleft, i.e. eustachian tube, middle ear, attic, aditus, antrum and mastoid air cells.

Aetiology

It is more common especially in infants and children of lower socio economic group. Typically, the disease follows viral infection of upper respiratory tract but soon the pyogenic organisms invade the middle ear.

Routes of Infection

1. Via eustachian tube. It is the most common route. Infection travels via the lumen of the tube or along subepithelial peritubal lymphatics. Eustachian tube in infants and young children is shorter, wider and more horizontal and thus may account for higher incidence of infections in this age group. Breast or bottle feeding in a young infant in horizontal position may force fluids through the tube into the middle ear and hence the need to keep the infant propped up with head a little higher. Swimming and diving can also force water through the tube into the middle ear.

2. Via external ear. Traumatic perforations of tympanic membrane due to any cause open a route to middle ear infection.

3. Blood-borne. This is an uncommon route.

Predisposing Factors

Anything that interferes with normal functioning of eustachian tube predisposes to middle ear infection. It could be:

1. Recurrent attacks of common cold, upper respiratory tract infections, and exanthematous fevers like measles, diphtheria, whooping cough.
2. Infections of tonsils and adenoids.
3. Chronic rhinitis and sinusitis.
4. Nasal allergy.
5. Tumours of nasopharynx, packing nose or nasopharynx for epistaxis.
6. Cleft palate.

Bacteriology. Most common organisms in infants and young children are Streptococcus pneumonia (30%), Hsaemophilus influenzae (20%) and Morexella catarrhalis (12%). Other organisms include streptococcus pyogenes, staphylococcus aureus and sometimes pseudomas aeroginosa. In about 18-20%, no growth is seen. Many of the strains of H. influenzae and Morexella catarrhalis are b-lactamase producing.

Pathology and Clinical Features

The diseases runs through the following stages:

1. Stage of tubal occlusion
2. Stage of pre-suppuration
3. Stage of suppuration
4. Stage of resolution or complication

1. Stage of tubal occlusion. Oedema and hyperaemia of nasopharyngeal end of eustachian tube, blocks the tube, leading to absorption of air and negative intratympanic pressure. There is retraction of tympanic membrane with some degree of effusion in the middle ear but fluid may not be clinically appreciable.

Symptoms. Deafness and earache are the two symptoms but they are not marked. There is generally no fever.

Signs. Tympanic membrane is retracted with handle of malleus assuming a more horizontal position, prominence of lateral process of malleus and loss of light reflex. Tuning fork tests show conductive deafness.

2. Stage of pre-suppuration. If tubal occlusion is prolonged, pyogenic organisms invade tympanic cavity causing hyperaemia of its lining. Inflammatory exudate appears in the middle ear. Tympanic membrane becomes congested.

Symptoms. There is marked earache which may disturb sleep and is of throbbing nature. Deafness and tinnitus are also present, but complained only by adults. Usually, child runs high degree of fever and is restless.

Signs. To begin with, there is congestion of pars tensa. Leash of blood vessels appear along the handle of malleus and at the periphery of tympanic membrane imparting it a cart-wheel appearance. Later, whole of tympanic membrane including pars flaccida becomes uniformly red. Tuning fork tests will again show conductive type of hearing loss.

3. Stage of suppuration. This is marked by formation of pus in the middle ear and to some extent in mastoid air cells. Tympanic membrane starts bulging to the point of rupture.

Symptoms. Earache becomes excruciating. Deafness increases, child may run fever of 102-103°F. This may be accompanied by vomiting and even convulsions.

Signs. Tympanic membrane appears red and bulging with loss of landmarks. Handle of malleus may be engulfed by the swollen and protruding tympanic membrane and may not be discernible. A yellow spot may be seen on the tympanic membrane where rupture is imminent. In pre-antibiotic era, one could see a nipple-like protrusion of tympanic membrane with a yellow spot on its summit. Tenderness may be elicited over the mastoid antrum.

X-rays of mastoid will show clouding of air cells because of exudate.

4. Stage of resolution. The tympanic membrane ruptures with release of pus and subsidence of symptoms. Inflammatory process begins to resolve. If proper treatment is started early or if the infection was mild, resolution may start even without rupture of tympanic membrane.

Symptoms. With evacuation of pus, earache is relieved, fever comes down and child feels better.

Signs. External auditory canal may contain blood tinged discharge which later becomes mucopurulent. Usually, a small perforation is seen in antero-inferior quadrant of pars tensa.Hyperaemia of tympanic membrane begins to subside with return to normal colour and landmarks.

5. Stage of complication. If virulence of organism is high or resistance of patient poor, resolution may not take place and disease spreads beyond the confines of middle ear. It may lead to acute mastoiditis, subperiosteal abscess, facial paralysis, labyrinthitis, petrositis, extradural abscess, meningitis, brain abscess or lateral sinus thrombophlebitis.

Treatment

1. Antibacterial therapy. It is indicated in all cases with fever and severe earache. As the most common organisms are Strept. pneumoniae and H. influenzae, the drugs which are effective in acute otitis media are ampicillin (50 mg/kg/day in 4 divided doses), amoxicillin (40 mg/kg/day in 3 divided doses). Those allergic to these penicillins can be given cefaclor, co-trimoxazole or erythromycin. In cases where beta-Iactamase-producing H. influenzae or Moraxella catarrhalis are isolated, antibiotics like amoxicillin-clavulanate, augmentin, cefuroxime axetil or cefixime may be used. Antibacterial therapy must be continued for a minimum of 10 days, till tympanic membrane regains normal appearance and hearing returns to normal. Early discontinuance of therapy with relief of earache and fever, or therapy given in inadequate doses may lead to secretory otitis media and residual hearling loss.

2. Decongenstant nasal drops. Ephedrine nose drops (1% in adults and 0.5% in children) or oxymetazoline (Nasivion) or xylometazoline (Otrivin) should be used to relieve eustachian tube oedema and promote ventilation of middle ear.

3. Oral nasal decongestants. Psudoephedrine (Sudafed) 30 mg twice daily or a combination of decongestant and antihistaminic (Triominic) may achieve drops which are difficult to administer in children.

4. Analgesics and antipyretics. Paracetamol helps to relieve pain and bring down temperature.

5. Ear toilet. If there is discharge in the ear, it is dry-mopped with sterile cotton buds and a wick moistened with antibiotic may be inserted.

6. Dry local heat. It helps to relieve pain.

7. Myringotomy. It is incising the drum to evacuate pus and is indicated when (a) drum is bulging and there is acute pain, (b) there is an incomplete resolution despite antibiotics when drum remains full with persistent conductive deafness, (c) there is persistent effusion beyond 12 weeks.

All cases of acute suppurative otitis media should be carefully followed till drum membrane returns to its normal appearance and conuctive deafness disappears.

6

Otalgia (Earache)

Pain in the ear can be due to problems occurring locally in the ear or referred to it from remote areas.

A. Local Causes

1. External ear. Furuncle, impacted wax, otitis externa, otomycosis, myringitis bullosa, herpes zoster, and malignant neoplasms.

2. Middle ear. Acute otitis media, eustachian tube obstruction, mastoiditis, extradural abscess, aero-otitis media, and carcinoma middle ear.

B. Referred Causes

As ear receives nerve supply from Vth (auriculotemporal br.), IXth (tympanic br) and Xth (auricular br.) cranial nerves; and from C_2 (lesser occipital) and C_2 and C_3 (greater auricular), pain may be referred from these remote areas.

1. Via Vth cranial nerve

(a) *Dental.* Caries tooth, apical abscess, impacted molar, malocclusion.

(b) *Oral cavity.* Benign or malignant ulcerative lesions of oral cavity or tongue.

(c) *Temporomandibular joint disorders.* Bruxism, osteoarthritis, recurrent dislocation, ill-fitting denture.

(d) *Sphenopalatine neuralgia.*

2. Via IXth cranial nerve

(a) *Oropharynx.* Acute tonsillitis, peritonsillar abscess, tonsillectomy. Benign or malignant ulcers of soft palate, tonsil and its pillars.

(b) *Base of tongue.* Tuberculosis or malignancy.

(c) *Elongated styloid process.*

3. Via Xth cranial nerve. Malignancy or ulcerative lesion of: vallecula, epiglottis, larynx or laryngopharynx, oesophagus.

4. Via C_2 and C_3 spinal nerves. Cervical spondylosis, injuries of cervical spine, caries spine.

C. Psychogenic

When no cause has been discovered, pain may be functional in origin but the patient should be kept under observation with periodic re-evaluation.

Otalgia is a *symptom*. It is essential to find its cause before specific treatment can be instituted.

7

Allergic Rhinitis

It is an IgE-mediated immunologic response of nasal mucosa to air-borne allergens and is characterised by watery nasal discharge, nasal obstruction, sneezing and itching in the nose. This may also be associated with symptoms of itching in the eyes, palate and pharynx. Two clinical types have been recognised:

1. Seasonal. Symptoms appear in or around a particular season when the pollens of particular plant, to which the patient is sensitive, are present in the air.

2. Perennial. Symptoms are present throughout the year.

Aetiology

Inhalant allergens are often the cause. Pollen from the trees and grasses, mold spores, house dust, debris from insects or house mite are common offenders. Food allergy is rarely an important cause.

Genetic predisposition plays an important part. Chances of children developing allergy are 20% and 47% respectively, if one or both parents suffer from allergic diathesis.

Pathogenesis

Inhaled allergens produce specific IgE antibody in the genetically predisposed individuals. This antibody becomes fixed to the blood basophils or tissue mast cells by its Fc end. On subsequent exposure, antigen combines with IgE antibody at its Fab end. This reaction produces degranulation of the mast cells with release of several chemical mediators, some of which already exist in preformed state while others are synthesised afresh. These mediators are responsible for symptomatology of allergic disease. Depending on the tissues involved, there may be vasodilation, mucosal oedema, infiltration with eosinophils, excessive secretion from nasal glands or smooth muscle contraction. A "priming affect" has also been described, i.e. mucosa earlier sensitised to an allergen will react to smaller doses of subsequnt specific allergen. It also gets "primed" to other non-specific antigens to which patient was not exposed. Clinically, allergic response occurs in 2 phases:

(a) Acute or early phase. It occurs immediately within 5-30 minutes, after exposure to the specific allergen and consists of sneezing, rhinorrhoea nasal blockage and/or bronchospasm. It is due to release of vasoactive amines like histamine.

(b) Late or delayed phase. It occurs 2-8 hours after exposure to allergen without additional exposure. It is due to infiltration of inflammatory cellseosinophils, neutrophils, basophil, monocytes and CD_4 +T cells at the site of antigen deposition causing swelling, congestion, thick secretion. In the event of repeated or continuous exposure to allergen, acute phase symptomatology overlaps the late phase.

Clinical Features

There is no age or sex predilection. It may start in infants as young as 6 months or older people. Usually the onset is at 12-16 years of age.

The cardinal symptoms of seasonal nasal allergy include paroxysmal sneezing, 10-20 sneezes at a time, nasal obstruction, watery nasal discharge and itching in the nose. Itching may also involve eyes, palate or pharynx. Some may get bronchospasm. The duration and severity of symptoms may vary with the season.

Symptoms of perennial allergy are not so severe as that of the seasonal type. They include frequent colds, persistently stuffy nose, loss of sense of smell due to mucosal oedema, postnasal drip, chronic cough and hearing impairment due to eustachian tube blockage or fluid in the middle ear.

Signs of allergy may be seen in the nose, eyes, ears, pharynx or larynx.

Nasal signs include transverse nasal crease a black line across the middle of dosrum of nose due to constant upward rubbing of nose simulating a salute (allergic salute), pale and oedematous nasal mucosa which may appear bluish. Turbinates are swollen. Thin, watery or mucoid discharge is usually present.

Ocular signs include oedema of lids, congestion and cobble-stone appearance of the conjunctiva dark circles under the eyes (allergic shiners).

Otologic signs include retracted tympanic membrane or serious otitis media as a result of eustachian tube blockage.

Pharyngeal signs include granular pharyngitis due to hyperplasia of submucosal lymphoid tissue. A child with perennial allergic rhinitis may show all the features of prolonged mouth breathing as seen in adenoid hyperplasia.

Laryngeal signs include hoarseness of voice and oedema of the vocal cords.

Diagnosis

A detailed history and physical examination is helpful, and also gives clues to the possible allergen. Other causes of nasal stuffiness should be excluded.

Investigations

1. *Total and differential count.* Peripheral eosinophilia may be seen but is an inconsistent finding.
2. *Nasal smear* shows large number of eosinophils in allergic rhinitis. Nasal smear should be taken at the time of clinically active disease or after nasal challenge test. Nasal eosinophilia is also seen in certain

nonallergic rhinitis, e.g. NARES (nonallergic rhinitis with eosinophilia syndrome).

3. *Skin tests* help to identify specific allergen. They are prick, scratch a intradermal tests.
4. *Radioallergosorbent test (RAST)* is an invitro test and measures specific IgE antibody concentration in the patient's serum.
5. *Nasal provocation test.* A crude method is to challenge the nasal mucosa with a small amount of allergen placed at the end of a toothpick and asking the patient to sniff into each nostril and to observe if allergic symptoms are reproduced. More sophisticated techniques are available now.

Complications

Nasal allergy may cause:

1. Recurrent sinusitis because of obstruction to the sinus ostia.
2. Nasal polypi.
3. Serous otitis media.
4. Orthodontic problems and other ill effects of prolonged mouth breathing especially in children.
5. Bronchial asthma. Patients of nasal allergy have four times more risk of developing bronchial asthma.

Treatment

Treatment can be divided into:

1. Avoidance of allergen
2. Treatment with drugs
3. Immunotherapy

1. Avoidance of allergen. This is most successful if the antigen involved is single. Removal of a pet from the house, encasing the pillow or mattress with plastic sheet, change of place of work or sometimes change of job may be required. A particular food article to which the patient is found allergic can be eliminated from the diet.

2. Treatment with drugs.

(a) *Antihistaminics.* They control rhinorrhoea, sneezing and pruritis. All antihistaminics have the side effects of drowsiness; some more than the other. The dose and type of the antihistaminic has to be individualised. If one antihistaminic is not effective, another may be tried from a different class.

(b) *Sympathomimetic drugs (oral or topical).* Alpha-adrenergic drugs constrict blood vessels and reduce nasal congestion and oedema. They also cause CNS stimulation and are often given in combination with antihistaminics to counteract drowsiness. Pseudoephedrine and phenyl-propanolamine are often combined with antihistamanics for oral administration.

Topical use of sympathomimetic drugs cause nasal decongestion. Phenylephrine, oxymetazoline and xylometazoline are often used to relieve nasal obstruction, but are notorious to cause severe rebound congestion. Patient resorts to using more and more of them to relieve nasal obstruction. This vicious cycle leads to rhinitis medicamentosa.

(c) *Corticosteroids.* Oral corticosteroids are very effective in controlling the symptoms of allergic rhinitis but their use should be limited to acute episodes which have not been controlled by other measures. They have several systemic side effects.

Topical steroids such as beclomethasone dipropionate, budesomide, flunisolide acetate fluticasone and mometasone inhibit recruitment of inflammatory cells into the nasal mucosa and suppress late-phase allergic reaction, are used as aerosols and are very effective in the control of symptoms. They have also been used in rhinitis medicamentosa while withdrawing topical use of decongestant nasal drops. Topical steroids have fewer systemic side effects but their continuous use may cause mucosal atrophy and even septal perforation. It is wise to break their use for 1-2 weeks every 2-3 months. They may promote growth of fungus.

(d) *Sodium chromoglycate.* It stabilises the mast cells and prevents them from degranulation despite the formation of 19B-antigen complex. It is used as 2% solution for nasal drops or spray or as an aerosol powder. It is useful both in seasonal and perennial allergic rhinitis.

3. Immunotherapy.

Immunotherapy or hyposensitisation is used when drug treatment fails to control symptoms or produces intolerable side effects. Allergen is given in gradually increasing doses till the maintenance dose is reached. Immunotherapy suppresses the formation of 19B. It also raises the titre of specific IgG antibody. Immunotherapy has to be given for a year or so before significant improvement of symptoms can be noticed. It is discontinued if uninterrupted treatment for 3 years shows no clinical improvement.

8

Epistaxis

Bleeding from inside the nose is called epistaxis. It is fairly common and is seen in all age groups children, adults and older people. It often presents as an emergency. Epistaxis is a sign and not a disease per se and an attempt should always be made to find any local or constitutional cause.

Blood Supply of Nose

Nose is richly supplied by both the external and internal carotid systems, both on the septum and the lateral walls.

Nasal Septum

Internal Carotid System

(a) Anterior ethmoidal artery.
(b) Posterior ethmoidal artery.
} Branches of ophthalmic artery

External Carotid System

(a) Sphenopalatine artery (branch of maxillary artery), gives nasopalatine and posterior nasal septal branches.

(b) Septal branch of greater palatine artery (Br. of maxillary artery).

(c) Septal branch of superior labial artery (Br. of facial artery).

Lateral Wall

Internal Carotid System

(a) Anterior ethmoidal	Branches of
(b) Posterior ethmoidal	ophthalmic artery

External Carotid System

(a) Posterior lateral nasal branches -> From sphenopalatine artery

(b) Greater palatine artery -> From maxillary artery

(c) Nasal branch of anterior superior dental -> From infraorbital branch of maxillary artery

(d) Branches of facial artery to nasal vestibule

Little's Area

It is situated in the anterior inferior part of nasal septum, just above the vestibule. Four arteries—anterior ethmoidal, septal branch of superior labial, septal branch of sphenopalatine and the greater palatine, anastomose form a vascular plexus called "Kiesselbach's plexus". This area is exposed to the drying effect of inspiratory current and to finger nail trauma, and is the usual site for epistaxis in children and young adults.

Retrocolumellar vein. This vein runs vertically downwards just behind the columella, crosses the floor of nose and joins venous plexus on the lateral nasal wall. This is a common site of venous bleeding in young people.

Causes of Epistaxis

They may be divided into:

A. Local, in the nose or nasopharynx.

B. General.

C. Idiopathic.

A. Local Causes

Nose

1. *Trauma.* Finger nail trauma, injuries of nose, intranasal surgery, fractures of middle third of face and base of skull, hard-blowing of nose, violent sneeze.

2. *Infections.*

   Acute: Viral rhinitis, nasal diphtheria, acute sinusitis.

   Chronic: All ernst-forming diseases, e.g.atrophic rhinitis, rhinitis sicca, tuberculosis, syphilis septal perforation, granulomatous lesion of the nose, e.g. rhinosporodiosis.

3. *Foreign bodies.*

   Non-living: Any neglected foreign body, rhinolith.

   Living: Maggots leeches.

4. *Neoplasms of nose and paranasal sinuses.*

   Benign: Haemangioma, papilloma.

   Malignant: Carcinoma or sarcoma.

5. *Atmospheric changes.* High altitudes, sudden decompression (Caisson's disease).

6. *Deviated nasal septum.*

Nasopharynx

1. Adenoiditis
2. Juvenile angiofibroma
3. Malignant tumours

B. General Causes

1. *Cardiovascular system.* Hypertension, arteriosclerosis, mitral stenosis, pregnancy (hypertension and hormonal).
2. *Disorders of blood and blood vessels.* Aplastic anaemia, leukaemia, thrombocytopenic and vascular purpura, haemophilia, Christmas disease, scurvy, vitamin K deficiency, hereditary haemorrhagic telangectasia.
3. *Liver disease.* Hepatic cirrhosis (deficiency of factorII, VII, IX & X).
4. *Kidney disease.* Chronic nephritis.
5. *Drugs.* Excessive use of salicylates and other analgesics (as for joint pains or headaches), anticoagulant therapy (for heart disease).
6. *Mediastinal compression.* Tumours of mediastinum (raised venous pressure in the nose).

7. *Acute general infection.* Influenza, measles, chickenpox, whooping cough, rheumatic fever, infectious mononucleosis, typhoid, pneumonia, malaria, dengue fever.
8. *Vicarious menstruation* (epistaxis occurring at the time of menstruation).

C. Idiopathic

Many times the cause of epistaxis is not clear.

Sites of Epistaxis

1. *Little's area.* In 90% cases of epistaxis, bleeding occurs from this site.
2. *Above the level of middle turbinate.* Bleeding from above the middle turbinate and corresponding area on the septum is often from the anterior and posterior ethmoidal vessels (internal carotid system).
3. *Below the level of middle turbinate.* Here bleeding is from the branches of sphenopalatine artery. It may be hidden, lying lateral to middle or inferior turbinate and may require infrastructure of these turbinates for localisation of the bleeding site and placement of packing to control it.
4. *Posterior part of nasal cavity.* Here blood flows directly into the pharynx.
5. *Diffuse.* Both from septum and lateral nasal wall. This is often seen in general systemic disorders and blood dyscrasias.
6. Nasopharynx.

Classification of Epistaxis

Anterior Epistaxis

When blood flows out from the front of nose with the patient in sitting position.

Posterior Epistaxis

Mainly the blood flows back into the throat. Patient may swallow it and later have a "coffee coloured" vomitus. This may erroneously be diagnosed as haematemesis.

The differences between the two types of epistaxis are tabulated herewith.

Management

In any case of epistaxis, it is important to know:

1. Mode of onset.
2. Duration and frequency of bleeding.
3. Amount of blood loss.
4. Side of nose from where bleeding is occurring.
5. Whether bleeding is of anterior or posterior type.
6. Any known bleeding tendency in the patient or family.
7. History of known medical ailment (hypertension, leukaemias, mitral valve disease, cirrhosis, nephritis).
8. History of drug intake (analgesics, anticoagulant, etc.)

First Aid

Most of the time, bleeding occurs from the Little's area and can be easily controlled by pinching the nose with thumb and index finger for about 5 minutes. This compresses the vessels of the Little's area. In Trotter's method patient is made to sit, leaning a little forward over a basin to spit any blood, and breathe quietly from the mouth. Cold compresses should be applied to the nose to cause reflexi vasoconstriction.

Cauterisation

This is useful in anterior epistaxis when bleeding point has been located. The area is first anaesthetised and the bleeding point cauterised with a bead of silver nitrate or coagulated with electrocautery.

Anterior Nasal Packing

In cases of active anterior epistaxis, nose is cleared of blood clots by suction and attempt is made to localise the bleeding site. In minor bleeds, from the accessible sites, cauterisation of the bleeding area can be done. If bleeding is profuse and/or the site of bleeding is difficult to localise, anterior packing should be done. For this, use a ribbon gauze soaked with liquid paraffin. About 1 metre gauze (2.5 cm wide in adults and 12 mm in children) is required for each nasal cavity. First, few centimetres of gauze are folded upon itself and inserted along the floor, and then the whole nasal cavity is packed tightly by layering the gauze from floor to the roof and from before backwards. Packing can also be done in vertical layers from back to the front. One or both cavities may need to be packed. Pack can be removed after 24 hours if bleeding has stopped. Sometimes, it has to be kept for 2 to 3 days; in that case, systemic antibiotics should be given to prevent sinus infection and toxic shock syndrome.

Posterior Nasal Packing

It is required for patients bleeding posteriorly into the throat. A postnasal pack is first prepared by tying three silk ties to a piece of gauze rolled into the shape of a cone. A rubber catheter is passed through the nose and its end brought out from the mouth. Ends of the silk threads are tied to it and catheter withdrawn from nose. Pack, which follows the silk thread, is now guided into the nasopharynx with the index finger. Anterior nasal cavity is now packed and silk threads tied over a dental roll. The third silk thread is cut short and allowed to hang in the oropharynx. It helps in easy removal of the pack later. Patients requiring postnasal pack should always be hospitalised. Instead of postnasal pack, a Folley's catheter can also be used. The bulb is inflated with saline and pulled forward so that choana is blocked and then an anterior nasal pack is kept in the usual manner. These days nasal balloons are also available. A nasal balloon has two bulbs, one for the postnasal space and the other for nasal cavity.

Endoscopic Cautery

Posterior bleeding point can sometimes be better located with an endoscope. It can be coagulated with suction cautery. Local anaesthesia with sedation may be required.

Elevation of Mucoperichondrial Flap and SMR Operation

In case of persistent or recurrent bleeds from the septum, just elevation of mucoperichondrial flap and then repositioning it back helps to cause fibrosis and constrict blood vessels. SMR operation can be done to achieve the same result or remove any septal spur which is sometimes the cause of epistaxis.

Ligation of Vessels

(a) *External carotid.* When bleeding is from the external carotid system and the conservative measures have failed, ligation of external carotid artery above the origin of superior thyroid artery should be done. It is avoided these days in favour of embolisation or ligation of more peripheral branches.

(b) *Maxillary artery.* Ligation of this artery is done in uncontrollable posterior epistaxis. Approach is via Caldwell- Luc operation. Posterior wall of maxillary sinus is removed and the maxillary artery or its branches are blocked by applying clips.

Endoscopic ligation of the maxillary artery can also be done through nose.

(c) *Ethmoidal arteries.* In anterosuperior bleeding above the middle turbinate, not controlled by packing, anterior and posterior ethmoidal arteries which supply this area, can be ligated. The vessels are exposed in the medial wall of the orbit by an external ethmoid incision.

General Measures in Epistaxis

1. Make the patient sit up with a back rest and record any blood loss taking place through spitting or vomiting.

2. Reassure the patient. Mild sedation should be given.
3. Keep check on pulse, blood preasure and respiration.
4. Maintain haemodynamics. Blood transfusion may be required.
5. Antibiotics may be given to prevent sinusitis, if pack is to be kept beyond 24 hours.
6. Intermittent oxygen may be required in patients with bilateral packs because of increased pulmonary resistance from nasopulmonary reflex.
7. Investigate and treat the patient for any underlying local or general cause.

Hereditary haemorrhagic telangectasia: It occurs on the anterior part of nasal septum and is the cause of recurrent bleeding. It can be treated by using Argon, KTP or Nd: YAG laser. The procedure may require to be repeated several times in a year as telangectasia recurs in the surrounding mucosa. Some cases require septodermoplasty where anterior part of septal mucosa is excised and replaced by a split skin graft.

9

Chronic Sinusitis

Chronic Sinusitis in General

Sinus infection lasting for months or years is called chronic sinusitis. Most important cause of chronic sinusitis is failure of acute infection to resolve.

Pathophysiology

Acute infection destroys normal ciliated epithelium impairing drainage from the sinus. Pooling and stagnation of secretions in the sinus invites infection. Persistence of infection causes mucosal changes, such as loss of cilia, oedema and polyp formation, thus continuing the vicious cycle.

Pathology

In chronic infections, process of destruction and attempts at healing proceed simultaneously. Sinus mucosa becomes thick and polypoidal (hypertrophic sinusitis) or undergoes atrophy (atrophic sinusitis). Surface epithelium may show desquamation, regeneration or metaplasia. Submucosa is infiltrated with lymphocytes and plasma cells and may show microabscesses, granulations, fibrosis or polyp formation.

Bacteriology

Mixed aerobic and anaerobic organisms are often present.

Clinical Features

Clinical features are often vague and similar to those of acute sinusitis but of lesser severity. Purulent nasal discharge is the commonest complaint. Foul-smelling discharge suggests anaerobic infection. Local pain and headache are often not marked except in acute exacerbations. Some patients complain of nasal stuffiness and anosmia.

Diagnosis

1. X-ray of the involved sinus may show mucosal thickening or opacity.
2. X-rays after injection of contrast material may show soft tissue changes in the sinus mucosa.
3. CT scan is particularly useful in ethmoid and sphenoid sinus infections and has replaced studies with contrast materials.

Treatment

It is essential to search for underlying aetiological factors which obstruct sinus drainage and ventilation. A work-up for nasal allergy may be required. Culture and sensitivity of sinus discharge helps in the proper selection of an antibiotic.

Initial treatment of chronic sinusitis is conservative, including antibiotics, decongestants, antihistaminics and sinus irrigations. More often, some form of surgery is required either to provide free drainage and ventilation or radical surgery to remove all irreversible diseases so as to provide wide drainage or to obliterate the sinus.

Recently, endoscopic sinus surgery is replacing radical operations on the sinuses and provides good drainage and ventilation. It also avoids external incisions.

10

Acute Tonsillitis

Primarily, the tonsil consists of (a) surface epithelium which is continuous with the oropharyngeal lining; (b) crypts which are tubelike invaginations from the surface epithelium; and (c) the lymphoid tissue. Acute infections of tonsil may involve these components and are thus classified as:

1. *Acute catarrhal or superficial tonsillitis.* Here tonsillitis is a part of generalised pharyngitis and is mostly seen in viral infections.
2. *Acute follicular tonsillitis.* Infection spreads into the crypts which become filled with purulent material, presenting at the openings of crypts as yellowish spots.
3. *Acute parenchymatous tonsillitis.* Here tonsil substance is affected. Tonsil is uniformly enlarged and red.
4. *Acute membranous tonsillitis.* It is a stage ahead of acute follicular tonsillitis when exudation from the crypts coalesces to form a membrane on the surface of tonsil.

Aetiology

Acute tonsillitis not only affects school-going children, but also adults. It is rare in infants and in persons who are above 50 years of age.

Haemolytic streptococcus is the most commonly infecting organism. Other causes of infection may be staphylococci, pneumococci or H. influenzae. These bacteria may primarily infect the tonsil or may be secondary to a viral infection.

Symptoms

The symptoms vary with severity of infection. The predominant symptoms are:

1. *Sore throat.*
2. *Difficulty in swallowing.* The child may refuse to eat anything due to local pain.
3. *Fever.* It may vary from 38 to 40°C and may be associated with chills and rigors. Sometimes, a child presents with an unexplained fever and it is only on examination that an acute tonsillitis is discovered.
4. *Earache.* It is either referred pain from the tonsil or the result of acute otitis media which may occur as a complication.
5. *Constitutional symptoms.* They are usually more marked than seen in simple pharyngitis and may include headache, general body aches, malaise and constipation. There may be abdominal pain due to mesenteric lymphadenitis simulating a clinical picture of acute appendicitis.

Signs

1. Often the breath is foetid and tongue is coasted.
2. There is hyperaemia of pillars, soft palate and uvula.
3. Tonsils are red and swollen with yellowish spots of purulent material presenting at the opening of crypts *(acute follicular tonsillitis)* or there may be a whitish membrane on the medial surface of tonsil which can be easily wiped away with a swab (*acute membranous tonsillitis*). The tonsils may be enlarged and congested so much so that they almost meet in the midline along with some oedema of the uvula and soft palate (*acute parenchymatous tonsillitis*).

4. The jugulodigastric lymph nodes are enlarged and tender.

Treatment

1. Patient is put to bed and encouraged to take plenty of fluids.
2. Analgesics (Aspirin or paracetamol) are given according to the age of the patient to relieve local pain and bring down the fever.
3. *Antimicrobial therapy*. Most of the infections are due to streptococcus, and penicillin is the drug of choice. Patients allergic to penicillin can be treated with' erythromycin. Antibiotics should be continued for 7-10 days.

Complications

1. *Chronic tonsillitis* with recurrent acute attacks. This is due to incomplete resolution of acute infection. Chronic infection may persist in lymphoid follicles of the tonsil in the form of microabscesses.
2. *Peritonsillar abscess.*
3. *Parapharyngeal abscess.*
4. *Cervical abscess* due to suppuration of jugulodigastric lymph nodes.
5. *Acute otitis media*. Recurrent attacks of acute otitis media may coincide with recurrent tonsillitis.
6. *Rheumatic fever*. Often seen in association with tonsillitis due to Group A beta-haemolytic streptococci.
7. *Acute glomerulonephritis*. Rare these days.
8. *Subacute bacterial endocarditis*. Acute tonsillitis in a patient with valvular heart disease may be complicated by endocarditis. It is usually due to streptococcus viridans infection.

11

What is Asthma?

Bronchial asthma, commonly called asthma, consists of repeated attacks of breathlessness and wheezing. When the patient is not in an attack, he feels normal. When an asthma patient comes in contact with an allergic substance, it behaves, as an antigen and reacts with the corresponding antibodies already present in his body. The histamine and other substances liberated during the allergic reactions cause the following changes in the bronchi:

1. Bronchial muscles are constricted to the content of lessening the diameter (calibre) of the bronchi.
2. Mucous membrane of the bronchi gets swollen, which further restricts the lemen of the bronchi.
3. Secretions are poured out from the swollen mucous lining into the constricted lumen of the bronchi.

When the bronchi are constricted and they are full of secretions, the patient has difficulty in breathing and his breath has a wheezing sound in it, which is more on breathing out because the bronchi gets narrower.

Asthma is a disease of the larger and medium-sized airways of the lungs and there is obstruction of outflow of air from the lungs. Since enough air does not reach the lungs for the exchange of gases, there is hurried breathing to compensate it.

Cough is a frequent symptom in asthmatics. This occurs in order to throw out the excessive secretions produced in the lungs.

This is particularly so in those who have respiratory infection as well. Cough gets relieved by the same measures as breathlessness.

The airways of the asthmatics are over-reactive to pollens, air pollution, changes in temperature, physical excercise, etc., and they react strongly to those factors. Persons who are asthmatics find it extremely difficult to tolerate smoking or air-pollution. Smoke or strong fumes, smell of fresh paint, white-washing, house-dust, or dust from old files, or the opening of dusty almirahs or trunks cause symptoms in some patients.

Asthma patients are liable to some complications such as thoracic deformity in children, diminished growth, recurrent infection or pneumonia, chronic bronchitis and hyper-inflation of the lung tissues (emphysema).

12

Diagnosis of Asthma by Skin Test

If asthma is caused or, at least, suspected by some allergen, try to find out as to which of the allergens is the real causative factor and also what and when symptoms surfaced first; in which seasons symptoms aggravated. It is quite necessary to take a detailed history of the patient; taking into account the said points. One would be expected to undergo the following tests with the advise of a specialist.

Skin Tests

In order to detect presence of reagins (antibodies) which are present in the skin and blood, skin tests are called for. Union of antibody in the skin, with its corresponding antigen applied in the skin tests, causes the release either of histamine-like or histamine substance by the tissues and results in redness and a weal around the site.

Skin tests are performed with extracts of pollens, moulds, dusts, etc. While concluding or carrying out such tests, it must be ensured that extracts are processed in most appropriate method, are neither old, active or potent, have no pathogenic micro-organisms in them and have minimal amount of any antigen. The results will be more accurate and precise if the antigen extract retains more natural characteristics. When the extract is ready (after sterilization and stardization), skin tests are carried out either by :

- Scratch Test or
- Intracutaneous test

Scratch Test

Skin of the arm or forehand is cleansed and a series of superficial abrasion/scratches of about ¼ cm long are made either of the said parts. It should be ensured that scratches or abrasions are not made deep lest bleeding takes places. Now allergence extracts are applied over the sight (which has been scratched / abrased) and removed after 15-20 minutes from the skin, and reactions occuring at the test site are observed an interpreted on the basis of comparison with control tests. Control tests are made with diluents of the allergenic principle.

Intracutaneous Tests

About 0.02 ml of each of the sterile allergenic extracts is introduced into the skin by a syring but reactions, due to application of this technique, are often quite larger than the ones obtained from the scratch test and the results obtained may also vary. It is necessary to carry out such intracutaneous tests with much care and precision otherwise, in most cases, allergic reactions are most likely to surface though such tests are not painful and can be easily carried out with children who soon lose their apprehension. These skin tests are graded from 0-4 + depending upon the degree of redness and swelling produced. If there is a significant positive reaction, the same must correspond to and match with the clinical history of the patient recorded earlier.

Grading of Skin Tests

Grade, size of weal and size of redness can be determined from the following table

Grade	Size of Weal	Size of Redness
0	Same as control	Same as control
1+	2 times more than control	10-20 mm

2+	3 times more than the control	20-30 mm
3+	4 times more than the control	More than 30 mm
4+	5 times more than the control	More than 40 mm

Normally negative reactions point out to absence of antibody against the tested allergen but other considerations (such as use of weak, inadequate or deteriorated extracts) can account for negative reactions/absence of antibody. Skin tests are carried out for following:

1. **Grasses:** Such as Sorghum, Cenchrus, Cynoden and Pennisetum.
2. **Trees:** Morus, Putranjiva, Cassia Siamea, Eucalyptus, Kigelia, Melia, Prosopis, Salvadora and Ricinus.
3. **Weeds:** Ageraturm, Adhatoda, Asphodelons, Brassica, Argemone, Chenopodium Album, Xanthium, Parthenium, Dodonea, Artemesia, Amaranthus and Parthenium.
4. **Fungi:** Mucor, Phoma, Alternaria, Candida, Aspergillus Fumigatus, cladodosporium, Helminthosporium.
5. **Danders:** Cat, Horse, Dog.
6. **Dusts:** Wheat dust, House dust, Paper dust, Cotton dust.

13

Kinds of Asthma

Asthma is of the following kinds:

Intrinsic Asthma

This type of asthma develops due to some pre-existing disease, like certain part infection or existing disease like bronchitis. Such type of patients do not benefit from or respond to anti-allergic treatment and, thus, not easy to manage and control due to non-response factor. This variety occurs mostly in advance age.

Extrinsic Asthma

Extrinsic asthma usually and commonly occurs in earlier part of one's life and generally responds to anti-allergic medication and treatment. The underlying cause can be attributed to exposure to allergic agents like certain fungi, house dust, pollens etc. The patient has an inherited tendency when he gets exposed to the said allergens. Recurring bouts of rhinites (sneezing) and eczema could also be the pre-disposing and precipitatory cause to trigger an attack of asthma.

Exercise Induced Asthma

This type of asthma commonly occurs to those who take to physical exercise in the cold weather but, then all persons may be either partially or not, at all, affected or some may be having serious manifestations.

Problems relating to asthma can be easily managed in young adults, but extremely difficult to mange in case of the elderly and small children.

Potential Asthmatic Patients

Following situations and type of persons could be termed as potential customers to imbibe asthma.

- Those who generally suffer from some sort of throat affection and there is recurrence of symptoms relating thereto.
- Those having a family history of asthma.
- Persons who often suffer from bouts of sneezing, especially at the change of season.
- Persons experiencing coughs at the change of season.
- Those living in polluted environments and whose houses are dark, damp, filthy, where standard of personal hygiene is appallingly poor and where sun rays cannot enter.
- Persons working in cloth mills, chemical factories, flour mills, paint and varnish factories, coal miners, labourers who work in stone quarries.
- Persons who easily get breathless even after a light exercise or due to change of season.
- Those who are sensitive to cold winds and develop breathing problem.
- Persons whose nose often remains blocked and, thus, have difficulty in breathing through nose.

There could be other situations/causes which may trigger an attack of asthma.

It is generally held that childhood eczema or development of sneezing in the grown up stage may manifest in the form of asthma. A child may inherit allergy but not a specific manifestation of allergy, that is allergy factor may be inherited but not the type/kind of allergy from which either parent suffers. Asthma has been observed to run from one generation to another.

Causes of allergy

- House Dust and Mites

- Plant pollens
- Fungi
- Insects/Insect bites
- Food Articles
- Animals
- Changing weather conditions
- Chemicals, Paints, Insecticides, Pesticides, Fertilizers (Indutrial Plooution)
- Smoke and fly-ash
- Heredity

Some other precipitatory factors may be sudden, coincidental or situation-based or some may be even specific to a person only in a given situation but disappear as soon as the agonizing situation becomes non-existent.

Causes of Ashtma

Asthma By House Dust
Asthma By Plant Pollens
Asthma By Fungi
Asthma By Insects
Asthma By Animals

14

Treating Asthma by Drugs

Asthma is treated firstly, to remove or lessen its symptoms and agony, and secondly, to remove its cause as far as possible. It is better and desirable that both aspects be undertaken side by side. Let us first take the drug treatment of asthma.

As we have already seen, a patient of asthma during an attack has narrowing of the airways and excessive production of lung secretions. The narrowed airways make respiration and exchange of gases in the lungs difficult, so that the patient has less of the oxygen and more of carbon dioxide in his blood.

The excessive secretions can within a short while lead to infection in the lungs, as the secretions are the nutrients of the different kind of bacteria and they grow very fast on it.

Furthermore, since a patient having an attack of asthma breathes very fast, he loses lot of water in the air which he throws out, and so loses a lot of water from his body.

Treatment During an Attack

- If the attack is very severe and prolonged, leading to deficiency of oxygen in the blood, which can be clinically ascertained by looking for bluish tinge on the body, tongue or conjunctivae, then administration of oxygen through nose is called for.
- The narrowing of the airways has to be removed and production of excessive secretion stopped.

- If there are signs of infection in the lungs, appropriate antibiotics are to be given.
- If the patient is dehydrated, intravenous 5 per cent glucose-saline is to be given.

Let us take up these items in more detail. Giving of Theophylline tablets, 2 tablets twice or thrice a day, depending upon the age, weight and severity of the condition, proves very helpful. Theophylline-Retard or sustained action tablets are also available.

The simplest and the well-tried drug combination for causing dilatation of the airways is giving a tablet which contains ephedrine, aminophylline and phenobarbitone. This combination is available under different proprietory names such as Tedral, Franal etc. This can be repeated two or three times a day. For children, syrups are available containing this combination.

For most patients having mild or moderate attack of asthma, this proves very helpful and even adequate in itself. Some patients do complain of palpitation after taking these tablets, and older patients having high blood pressure have to take it in lesser quantities. Ephedrine in it can cause constipation and if the patient has some enlargment of the prostate, it can cause some difficulty in passing urine. But generally speaking, such tablets prove very efficacious.

Drugs like salbutamol (which are B-2 stimulators) have come into use lately. They specifically dilate the bronchial airways without excessively stimulating the heart, so that they do not usually lead to palpitation. These drugs come in the form of tablets, injections or aerosol inhalers. In combination with deriphylline, salbutamol tablets prove very useful.

In case there is a severe attack of asthma, deriphylline injection given intramuscularly or aminophylline with 5 per cent glucose intravenously, slowly in 5 to 10 minutes proves helpful. Aminophylline given through intravenous drip with 5 per cent glucose is very useful. An injection of adrenaline (1 : 1000 solution) ½ ml, given very slowly subcutaneously, is also effective in many cases.

Most patients usually need only this medication and care. But, at times, the symptoms increase or when an infection supervenes, extra care is needed. If bacterial infection is present in the respiratory passages and unless properly and adequately treated, bronchodilator drugs either exert diminished action or have no action at all, so that the patient keeps getting breathless. So, as far as possible, the causative organism must be identified, its sensitiveness to a drug found, and then the proper drug administered.

But in the majority of the cases, this is not possible either because of the lack of facilities or the procedure takes more time than a patient can afford. In such a situation, ampicillin has been found to be helpful: one or two capsules of 250 mg thrice a day for a week proves adequate; the dose and length of administration depends, however, upon the severity of infection.

If the attack of asthma is such that it is not controlled by the bronchodilator tablets, injections as well as the antibiotics, then the patient can be put on corticosteroids. These can be given as tablets or intramuscularly or in very severe cases, intravenously.

Treatment in Status Asthmaticus

If the patient has been in status asthmaticus (i.e., continuous and severe attack of asthma for more than 24 hours), it is important to keep in mind that he may also be dehydrated because of excessive loss of water from the lungs; by excessive perspiration and by omitting to take fluids while in an attack. Hence his fluid loss has to be replaced adequately. This besides restoring the fluid balance of the body, lessens the thickness of the tenacious sputum so that it is coughed out easily. In such a case, intravenous fluids are administered early, usually 3 to 5 litres in the first twenty-four hour period, and thereafter 3 litres daily until hydration is achieved. Fluids usually consist of 5 per cent dextrose in water; every second or third such fluid should contain sodium chloride, particularly if prolonged intravenous therapy in necessary, or if the patient is perspiring freely and he vomits or has diarrhoea. As th patient becomes hydrated and starts eating well, the intravenous administration of fluids can be curtailed.

A cyanosed patient of asthma in status asthmaticus is in need of oxygen which must be given. This can be given either through a catheter in the nose or through a ventri-mask or through a positive pressure breathing apparatus along with a bronchodilator; the last mode of therapy has proved to be more effective.

The use of expectorants in the management of asthma is one of the most important yet often neglected aspects of treatment. One of the best expectorants is potassium iodide; when it is tolerated poorly, other substances such as glyceral guiacolate and ammonium chloride may be useful. Water vapour also may be helpful in thinning bronchial secretions.

Patients with severe asthma become profoundly exhausted, lose sleep, experience increasing anxiety, and therefore, are in need of a tranquilliser, but is should be kept to a minimum, because excess of it can interfere with respiration.

Deaths from asthma can occur in spite of the antibiotics and steroids. These occur not only in older people who die of the complications of long-standing asthma, but also in younger people aged between 5 and 35 years. Majority of these deaths occur outside the hospital. These are due to the fact that the patient and his relations could not realise the severity of the situation.

A proper understanding of the patient's fears and anxieties and the allaying of these fears through sympathetic conversation helps asthma patients very much. The majority of these patients are prone to suggestion. It has been seen, time and again, that when a prescription is given or a line of treatment is started with the emphatic suggestion to the patient that this will definitely give relief, it decidedly works and the patient fulfils the expectations. Not only that, I have observed, that with whatever symptoms the patient looks better, produces a corresponding response and the hope given that "You will imporve still further", works miracle. Such an approach is helpful, but care must be taken because over-optimistic hopes, once shattered, cause more harm than good.

Aerosol Inhalers

Aerosol are the solid or liquid particles of a substance suspended in air. They are very small, less than a micron (1/1000 mm) in size.

Aerosol inhalers were used initially with bronchodilator drugs like Isoprenaline. But because this drug caused many side-effects such as palpitation and dizziness and some deaths too due to too frequent use, this mode of treatment fell into some disrepute.

With the availability of aerosol inhalers with salbutamol and corticosteroids, this form of treatment has now become very popular.

The technique of using the inhaler is as follows:

- Shake the inhaler. Remove the cap from its mouth-piece. Insert the mouth-piece in the lips and purse the lips tightly around it.
- Take one or two breaths with the inhaler in the mouth.
- Exhale completely, and then as you start inhaling, press the nozzle-button of the inhaler. Aerosol would go in the airways alongwith the air inhaled.
- Now remove the inhaler from the mouth. Keep the lips closed, and hold the breath as long as possible, then open the mouth.
- You can repeat the process and take one more does of aerosol from the inhaler. The dose that comes out each time on pressing the inhaler is equal and is measured.

Cortisone

Cortisone, the miracle drug, has provided renewed hopes to the patient suffering from very severe forms of allergies including asthma. This is a very potent drug and ought to be used in acute life-threatening situations. In asthma cases, cortisone can help patients where nothing else helps, but then it ought to be used only when everything else has been tried and has failed.

It is difficult to say which manifestation of allergy are helped the most, but it is the asthma patients who make maximum use of them.

Among the asthma patients, corticosteroids have provided the maximum and most-needed relief to those having status asthmaticus. Intramuscular or intravenous asministration abolishes symptoms in those patients in whom adrenaline or aminophylline have not been of much use. After corticosteroid administration, some of the patients who previously did no respond to adrenaline or aminophylline start responding can be resorted to. Gradually the corticosteroids can be tapered off and the patient can be put on other routine bronchodilators.

Short term use of corticosteroids has proved very helpful to those asthma patients who do not do well with the usual bronchodilators or to those who do not get adequate relief from them.

With the dosage and time for which these drugs are usually prescribed, no serious side effects or complications are observed. Complaints of general weakness or epigastric distress or diminished appetite are certainly not more than are encountered when patients are given ephedrine and aminophylline.

Acute attacks not responding to other routine measures, show excellent improvement in seasonal asthma cases. On the other hand, perennial asthmatic cases who have developed irreversible structural changes in the lungs, do not respond very well.

Care in Administration: The conditons generally forbid the use of cortisone are diabetes mellitus, pepticulcer, gastrointestinal bleeding, tuberculosis, psychosis, old age, chronic kidney disease, heart attack and significant hypertension. However, these contraindications are more relative than absolute. Long-term taking of corticosteroids may produce hairiness (hirsutism) over the face.

While corticosteroids are being taken, an acute infection in the body does not produce as much symptoms as it would do otherwise.

Hence, if the symptoms of an infection are even minor, a doctor ought to be consulted.

Upon discontinuation of the corticosteroids, or on a too rapid decrease dosage, some patients complain of tiring easily, weakness, nervousness, irritability, gastro-intestinal disturbances and occasional dizziness.

Cortisone Inhaler: In cases of intractable asthma where other medications have failed or have not provided adequater relief and cortisone tablets have to be taken, cortisonc inhaler reduces the need for the tablets. Since the inhaled cortisone acts locally in the lungs, it hardly produces any side-effects. The inhaler is needed to be used 3 to 4 times a day and provides appreciable relief.

Inhalations of cortisone on heavy dosage and for long periods can be lead to growth of fungi in the throat, causing soreness and discomfort. If it happens, the inhalations have to be stopped.

Antihistamines in Asthma

Antihistamines are not effective in the case of asthma in adults. They have no effect on bronchospasm; in fact, the symptoms sometimes get aggravated because of the drying up of the secretions and the subsequent difficulty in passing phlegm. Allergic cough in children, however, is helped by giving antihistamines along with a bronchodilator in cough mixture.

Any drug taken should be in consultation with your doctor.

15

Inhalation Devices You Can Use

Powder Inhaler

Powder Inhalers are devices that deliver a measured dose of medicine in a powdered form. The transparent Rotahaler is one such device. It uses a capsule to deliver the medicine and is very easy to use.

Spray Inhaler

The Spray Inhaler is the most widely used inhalation device in the world. It delivers a measured dose of medicine through a pressurised spray. To get the full benefit from a spray inhaler, it is essential to use it in a proper way.

Spacer

The spacer is a holding chamber which can be attached to the Spray Inhaler. It makes the Spray Inhaler easier to use and adds to its effectiveness.

Nebuliser

Nebulisers are used for giving higher doses of medication at times when breathing becomes very difficult. They are machines that transform the medicine into a fine mist, which can be breathed in by normal breathing, via a facemask or a mouthpiece. Nebulisers are usually used in hospitals and nursing homes, for the management of severe attacks.

16

Hiccough / Hiccup

Medically, the disease is also known as 'Singultus'. There is an abrupt involuntary lowering of the diaphragm and closure of sound-producing folds, at the upper end of the trachea, producing a characteristic sound when the breath is inspired (drawn in). Hiccups occurs repeatedly and almost in quick succession or the gap between two hiccups (paroxysmal period) is so short that the patient does not have any respite. In fact spasmodic contraction of the diaphragm (which is more often reflex) or mid-riff is the basic cause of hiccup which is a reflex from the kidney/liver/stomach etc. Since heart rests immediately over the diaphragm, so spasmodic contraction of it leads to repeated jerks on the heart; hence there is exhausation.

Hiccup is a serious disease due to dose affinity of heart and diaphragm, especially when the problem is associated with previous exhaustion and/or serious malady but the hiccup found in children and others is usually of hysterical nature (hysterical hiccup); hence is not that dangerous as spasmoitic hiccup(s).

General and traditional method, often practised is either to divert attention of the patient from episodes of hiccup or give water to be sipped only. I have seen certain cases improve instantaneously. About 5 years back I was staying with a business friend whose 18 year old girl had repeated paroxysms of exhausted; her eyes looking dangerously lachrymal and red. I suddenly entered her room and asked the young one to turn her back. When she turned her back, I blowed her back portion, within the shoulders, with a sudden jerking blow and, surprisingly, she breathed a sigh of relief and had no hiccups thereafter. It all implies that distraction of mind is necessary but may not always prove availing.

Homeopathic Treatment

Ginseng-Q: Should be used in all forms of hiccup (Give 5 drops with water)-may be repeated if attacks do not stop.

Cuprum Met / Cuprum Ars-6: If hiccup is accompanied with nausea, eructations, difficult breathing, or if drinking of water relieves hiccup.

Ignatia-6: When hiccup is caused after or followed by smoke, food or drink.

Carbo Veg-6: When caused by movement.

Lycopodium-30: When the tongue at one time is drawn in, and at another time extruded.

Cicuta-6: Hiccup with sound.

Cocculus-6: Hiccup and eructations, stabbing pain.

Nux Vom-3: If hiccup occurs, before meals are taken. Some people recommend water of green coconut or kernel inside the stone of palm fruit. Diet given should be in liquid and bland form.

Occasional paroxysms of hiccup, if short lived and abating quickly, should not cause any concern but prolonged attacks need to be treated, as some attacks are so quick and exhausting that the patient becomes nervous and cyanotic, breathing is also under strain, hence, in the later stage, there is no room for any complacent approach.

Croup

This is predominantly a children's disease when there is a stredor (deep, sharp sound) due to impeded breathing, constriction of chest and its capacity to expand and contract diminishes, face becomes pale, head tilts on one side and facial muscles benum. But all the above mentioned signs are not long-lasting. After a short while, there are convulsions and cramps in the whole body, and in grave situations breathing stops (asphaxia) and finally the patient dies of suffocation.

Children between the age of 3 months and 2 years are generally the victims, attacks mostly coming at night. Children who are extremely weak and are brought up under unhygienic and unhealthy environs, fall prey to this horrible disease.

Treatment

It mostly consists of pure air, water and food. Food must be served with high nutritional values. Health building tonics like Ostomalt, Cod Liver oil with malt extract, Adexoline drops etc may be given either along/with milk/or before or after milk, whenever the attack takes place; pat and sponge the child with hot or cold water, according to weather conditions. He may be given Ammonia to inhale 4-5 drops of. Tincture of Castor may be mixed with hot/ cold water. Homeopathic medicines like pot. Bromide (kali Bromide-30) or/and chlorum (chloral hydrate)-6 may be given with water; crude dose being 2-5gms of Pot Bromide and ½ -2gms of chloral hydrate. Before any medicine is given to child, it is advised that the child is never treated at home, rather he should be examined by a doctor so that there is no delay in proper treatment.

17

Cold and Coryza

Cold may affect the nose, throat as a result of which water may start running from the nose, there is headahe, chill, slight fever, aching all over the body and feeling of rundown condition. It is caused by exposure to cold, in any form, or entering a cool room, or going out in the open . Exposure to cold is the main cause. The patient feels rawness in the throat, nasal passages inflame due to congestion of its mucus lining, cough is hawked up with much difficulty; there being general restivity and disinclination to do any work. As a general rule, head, chest and throat should be wrapped so as to avoid further exposure to these parts.

Home Treatment

Aconite 30: Feverishness, sneezing, fear of death, constant chill, occasional shivering, general coldness of body, raw sensation or burning in the throat.

Arsenic Album-30: In spite of running of water, the nose is stuffed up or blocked discharge, is hot and acrid; general malaise and restlessness.

Allium Cepa 30: Useful when there is free, profuse and constant discharge of water from the nose, sneezing, on entering a warm room.

Kali Bichrom 6x (powder): When there is tenacious and sticky discharge which is difficult to expel; ulceration of nose, loss of sense of smell.

Ammon. Carb-6: Tip of nose is red and painful, ulcers in the nostrils, stuffing of nose at night, discharge is in the form of blood or mucus; bleeding from nose, while washing face in the morning.

Euphrasia-Q: There is profuse nasal secretion with repeated and tiring sneezing.

Pulsatilla-6: Discharge is thick and greenish yellow, loss of taste and smell, sense of suffocation in a warm room; disease due to heavy use of fats which the patient tolerates well.

Nux Vomica-6: Useful when running from nose has stopped but, despite that, the nose feels tightened up, bowels impacted and ineffectual urging to defecate, headache, dyspepsia.

Sepia-30: When there is catarrhal blockade of nose all the year round. More useful in chronic stage of the disease.

Allopathic Treatment

Tablet Actifed-one tablet twice/three times a day will stop running from the nose. The dose may be halved if there is drowsiness. Tablet Avil (25 mg) taken thrice daily will also abort flow from nose and also stop sneezing or a tablet of Cosavil-2/3 times daily—will also have similar effect but will also be useful in fever and body pain. Tablet Dristan is an all round medicine to control almost all the related symptoms of cold, mild cough, stuffing/running from nose, fever, body pain, and is more useful in chronic stage.

If nostrils get stuffed up, use Efcorlin Nasal drops (2-3 drops in each nostril) to clear blockade. It will also facilitate stuck up mucus in the nose so as to facilitate breathing.

Whatever the situation of cold, always take a 500 mg tablet of Vitamin-C (Sukrets or Celen) once a day to enhance general resistance to cold. In acute stage, the dose may be raised to 2 tablets a day. 10-20 drops of Benzoin compound mixed with hot water and inhaled at night will have all-round relief in relieving congestion in the entire respiratory tract; but exposure must be avoided.

Ayurvedic treatment

Mix garlic juice (5ml) with basil, 4 black peppers, a clove and honey (say 5 ml) will cure the disease or suck Vyoshaadi Vati or Marichaadi Vati or Sugar Candy or Mulethi.

Godanti Bhasma (400 mg), Ras Sindoor (150 or 200 mg) Praval Bhasma (100 mg) and Tankan Bhasma (100 mg) should be mixed. Garlic juice (10-15 ml) and equal quantity of honey is an all-round efficacious compound.

Use hot water in plenty, especially after or with meals. Sitoplaadi Churma (100 mg), Tanken Bhasma (200 mg), Mulethi (400 mg) should be mixed up with honey and taken 2-3 times daily. Nasal blockade can be removed by inserting shada Bindu Tail (3 drops in each nostril). It will also clear up sinus affections.

Tea with basil and garlic is also useful to soothe the agitated respiratory passage. In any case, avoid exposure to cold winds. Keep your head and chest fully wrapped with woolen garments/ coverings.

Cinnamon powder (500-800 mg) boiled in milk, 5 ml of clarified butter will provide relief in cold, if taken at bed time. But, should not be used by those who have bilious temperament or whose liver is sluggish. Bread of whole grams with clarified butter (ghee), followed by a glassful of lemon juice, mixed in hot water, will provide much strength and relief. It will reduce sneezing spells, clear nose and soothe the throat.

1 part purified (parched) borax, 5 parts liquourice powder, and 12 parts honey (1:5:12 ratio) should be mixed together so as to prepare a liquefied paste. Normal dose being 1 tsp for adults, ½ tsp for children, ¼ or ¼th tsp for infants three or four times daily will cure even protracted and inveterate cases of chronic asthma, cough, coryza, and even tonsillitis.

18

Weather Changes and Cough

Some patients are found to have their symptoms aggravated during peak days of winter season when dry cold winds blow, some suffer during rainy season or when the wind is pregnant with moisture, whereas, in some, summer days, especially dust raising winds cause cough. Such cases develop acute symptoms and when the weather changes, they improve but if the disease persists beyond 10-15 days or even after the congenial weather conditions have set, then the disease assumes a chronic form. Such types of cough have almost identical symptoms on each weather condition. Chnage of venue and environs often show encouraging results. Self-management is another option when it is not possible to change-over to more congenial environs.

Treatment of cough (Homeopathic)

This mostly is caused during rainy season. Phlegm is yellow, stickly, abundant and difficult to cough up. Try following medicines according to specific symptoms noted against each remedy.

Nat.Suplh 6: Is the leading remedy. Take 4 hourly doses a day. Avoid curd, whey, milk etc.

Aconite 6: Cough abates on lying down but aggravates on lying down on a side. Headache, constipation, chilliness, anxiety, fear of death, chest excited by cold blast, cough dry.

Calc.Carb 6: Dry cough, especially worse at bed-time.

Ipecac-30: Suffocating/spasmodic cough, difficult breathing, wheezing sound with sore throat or rattling noise due to accumulation of phlegm, pain in navel while cough, nausea or vomiting.

Antim Tart-30: Voice hoarse, dry cough, vomiting of food due to cough following food, mucus is liquid but difficult to expel, there is rattling of throat, between intervals of cough yawning takes place. Useful for young infants whose chest remains filled up with phlegm and there is a gurgling sound as the chest is filled up with phlegm. Nostrils are also blocked.

Bryonia-30: Pain in chest, tearing / sticking pain in head, on sides, cough convulses whole body, cough aggravated from exposure to cold draughts-worse in the morning or evening. At times cough is blood-tinged, with thin expectortion, cough aggravated while entering a cold room from a warm place/room, cough excited after drinking or eating. Cough abates while lying on the affected side.

Belladonna-200: Inflammation of larynx, dry cough at night; flushed face; pulse is quick and hard; face flushed, eyes bright; dry cough with choking or spasm, cold helps to moisten the cough and helps to bring up shreds of mucus; relief in cold air; cough more at night than during the day.

Nitric Acid 6

More useful in chronic cough; cough dry with melancholy, headache, debility, loss of appetite, heaviness at pit of stomach after eating; pain in stomach; sweating, insomnia, constipation, pain behind breast-bone; is said to be more useful when infection is acute and severe.

Ignatia-6: It is a specific remedy when anxiety, sudden shock or worry be the cause. More useful in nervous cough, caused by sudden bad news. Disturbed mental condition is the keynote: Also useful for cough of hysterics, spasm of wind-pipe, night's rest is disturbed by cough, tickling in throat aggravates cough.

Rumex-6: Aggravation in the morning or at night or exposure to cold wind. patient feels relieved when whole body is fully covered from head to feet. Cough is dry and constant which convulses the whole body.

Drosera-6: Cough is dry and rises from throat, there is constant pain and tickling sensation; there is often loss of voice; cough closely resembles whooping cough bouts; throat is scraped and, at times, sputum could be even blood-tinged, patient belches and vomits; there are occasional spasms of cough which are exhausting and tiring, aggravation of cough at time.

Causticum-6: Hoarse voice, dry, brazen cough-often leading to unconscious evacuations; aggravation while entering a warm room but abates after taking some cold drink; patient can bring the sputum upto throat but is unable to cough it out.

Spongia-6: Cough is dry, scraping, irritating and painful; suffocation; pain in chest, voice hoarse, due to spasm of windpipe, the patient finds it difficult to breathe. Cough ameliorates after drinking/eating.

Kali Bichrome-6: This is specific remedy when throat or chest is filled up with mucus but cannot be expelled due to its being sticky, tough, adhesive and tenacious; the patient exerts a lot more to bring up cough and if it comes up, at all, it would get stuck in the throat or adhere to lips; there is dizziness and vertigo due to constant coughing which brings up even blood. Aggravation after getting in the morning from bed and after meals. Asthmatics may try this remedy when windpipe and throat are filled up with phlegm (sticky and tenacious).

Phosphorus-30: Pain in chest, hoarse voice, dry cough with tickling in throat; sputum is frothy, rusty, saltish, purulent; cough aggravates due to laughing; talking or on reading—that is when utmost pressure is exerted on larynx and throat; voice is hoarse, throat painful, chest is also painful. Cough is dry.

Pulsatilla-30: Sputum is yellow or greenish, bitter in taste; accumulation of phlegm in chest causes suffocation; there is rattling noise in throat; sputum during day, but is bitter at night or when lying down; worse in closed room but better when coming in the open air.

In emergent situations, give Passiflora Incarnata-Q (15-30 drops in tepid water, preferably at bed time or at anytime during crisis period). It will soothe the agitated nerves, calm down cough spells and also induce sound sleep. Lobelia-Q or Senega-Q (5 drops mixed with water) may also meet demands of crisis stage.

When the situation is not possible to manage at home, at once seek medical help.

General

In my opinion steam inhalation is an excellent method to allay even emrgent situations. Steam will loosen cough and help sputum to expectorate, sooth and comfort throat, wind-pipe and lungs and remove congestion, if any. It will also remove nasal blood and, thus, facilitate respiration. After steam inhalation, there should be no exposure to cold winds or else the malady would assume more complex appearance. To make steam inhalation more effective, add ¼ tsp of Vicks Vaporub so as to derive quicker relief. No Homeo medicine should be served an hour before or after the process. After inhalation, whole mouth may be gently patted and rubbed with a small towel so as to improve blood circulation on/ around face.

Biochemic Treatment

There are 12 tissue/inorganic salts which are claimed to cure all the curable diseases. Major salts are : Calc. Flour; Calc.Phos, Ferrum Phos, Kali Mur, Kali Phos, Kali Sulph, Mag.Phos, Natrum Phos, Nat Sulph, Calc.Sulph and Silicea.All are used in 3, 6 or 12 potences. Silicea is generally used in 30 or 200. These medicines are prepared homeopathically also wherein 3, 6, 12, 30, 200 or higher potencies are used. Difference lies in preparatory method only, though effect and efficacy do not vary much.

Read carefully composition of following combination wherein more then three biochemic medicines have been combined so as to cover most of the symptoms. Biochemic preparations can be given either alone or in alteration with homoepathic medicines, if symptoms are not at variance. Biochemic combinations have been allotted specific numbers.

No-2 Asthma

Components: Kali Phos, Mag. Phog, Nat.Mur, Nat.Sulph

No-5 (Coryza)

Components: Fer.Phos, Kali Mur. Nat Mur, Kali Sulph

No-6 (Cough, Cold, Catarrh)

Components: Fer.Phos, Kali Mur. Magn. Phos, Nat Mur, Nut Sulph.

No-10 (Enlarged Tonsils)

Components: Clac. Phos, Fer. Phos, Kali Mur.

Allopathic Treatment

Any cough expectorant syrup (like Corex, Phensydyl, Dilosyn, Benadryl, etc.) will help to first loosen and then expectorate cough. Certain drowsiness or blurred vision may occur during the course of taking anyone of the above cough syrups; hence one should refrain from driving a vehicle operating a machine or while moving out. Usual dose is 5 ml (1 tsp) three times daily. It is claimed that the last dose, at bed time, if taken in hot water, will show better results, including sound sleep. In smokers' cough, Glycodin Terp Vasaka is still considered a choiced cough syrup.

Steam inhalation, as suggested earlier, may be had. If some infection is the cause, then anyone of the antibiotics like Septran D.S, Ciprafloxin 500 mg, 500 mg (each 12 hourly, that is a dose after 12 hours). Lorvas tab (one a day dose) is said to control allergic coughs but has to be continued for a long time.

Saline water gargles will provide much needed relief in throat infections, after which some throat pain may be applied locally.

Caution

It is specifically pointed out that the patient should seek advice of his doctor, in so far as dosage of a particular medicine and side effects thereof are concerned. More care and caution is needed in acute and emergent cases when routine medicines a well-tried formulation, cannot be ruled out. Hence, expert's advice is quite necessary. Infants and pregnant women, old and infirm persons also should never be treated by a layman, as they react to medicines more quickly than others.

It can be easily deduced that one or more than one medicine has been repeated in almost all the above-mentioned combinations, except Kali Phos, Calc.Phos and Kali Sulph which have not been repeated, except once. So, the combinations do not vary much and absence of a particular salt goes to prove that non-mentioned drug is a specific drug mentioned in a particular context.

Ayurvedic Treatment

If cough is caused due to Vaata (wind) vitiation, give Panchamrita Ras/Taalishaadi Choorna/Amritarnava Rasa 200 mg thrice daily with honey. Anyone of the medicines will help in expectoration of sputum. But first of all remove constipation.

When cough is caused due to vitiation of bile, pitta Kasantak Ras/Singhyadi Vati (dose-100mg/200mg/1 tsp respectively) may be taken, but no medicine should be mixed, rather taken independently. If Praval Pishthi or Praval Bhasma is also added to any one of the above compositions (dose 400 mg to 1 gm), it will still be more beneficial. It will modify ill effects of bile, phlegm and heat also.

For cough, aggravated by phlegm vitiation, it is necessary to control expectoration. Give Kasa Kuthar Ras (100 mg) with milk, which has been fortified with Panchkole, Swachhand Bhairav Ras (200 mg) with honey; Shringa Bhasma/Krishnaabhra Bhasam/Ras Sindoor/Tankan Bhasm (50-100mg) may also be mixed with above-mentioned medicines.

Vasarishta/Pippalyasava/Kankasava (5-10 ml with water) may be given after each meal.

In tubercular cough Agastya Haritaki (5-10 ml in water) with goat's milk is quite beneficial. Laxmi vilas ras can also be used with medicines suggested under phlegmatic cough.

Light food, fresh air, airy and ventilated house, goat's milk, dried dates boiled in milk, fruit juice of non-citrus fruits, avoid all throat irritants, cold water, smoking, coitus, excessive exertion, or any exercise that causes dyspnoea/panting.

19

Respiratory Infection and Diarrhoea

Hygiene of body, food items should be proper and if it is a case of a child, this should be best. A little exposure of harmful bacteria may lead to several disorders and complications.

Diarrhoea in Children

Diarrhoea in children can be fatal due to loss of water and salts (electrolytes) from the body via stools. The risk is more in young children as their body is small, thus the loss is very fast and becomes life threatening.

Diarrhoea as such leaves the child not merely dehydrated but also malnourished. It makes her more prone to other diseases.

Thus, it is important that every child gets very good care during episodes of diarrhoea.

The focus of care is essentially on two things:

1. Prevent dehydration and replace lost fluids and salts at the earliest.
2. Maintain good nutrition for the child.

As soon as the child starts having loose motions, don't wait for anything. Immediately start giving some home available fluids, e.g. daal (pulse) water, lassi, rice water, coconut water, light tea, lemon-sugar shikanji or simply plain water. You can also fetch a packet of Oral Rehydration Salts (ORS) from the nearest health facility (or even from chemist's shop). Follow the instruction given on the packet to make it. Generally, one packet is to be dissolved in one litre of safe drinking water.

For each stool passed, give 200 ml of ORS to the child or as much as the child can drink comfortably. Give small, frequent sips in between also. Contact a health worker for further advise.

This advise must be sought as soon as possible if the child has any one of the following symptoms:

- Blood /mucus in stool
- Child is having excessive vomiting.
- Child is not getting better with ORS
- Child is not passing urine

Normal feeding must be continued during diarrhoea. It simply means a breast fed child must be continued on breast feeds. A child who has been on semi solid/solid diet also must be given this food during diarrhoeal episode. The only change you can make is to keep the spices and chillies low in the food.

Once a child recovers from diarrhoea, give her/him extra food for atleast one week.

Do remember that most of the diarrhoeal episodes are self limiting and get well on their own, without any medicines. Infact, don't give any anti diarrhoeal medicines to the child on your own. Seek the help of a health worker because self medication can be dangerous in general and in diarrhoea in particular.

Acute Respiratory Infections in Children (Common Cold; Pneumonia)

Acute Respiratory Infections (ARIs) claim lives of about 1 million (10 lakh) children of less than 5 year of age every year, in India.

It is important to take some precautions if your child gets an attack of ARI.

A child with common cold often becomes irritated and refuses the feeds. She/he often has fever, running or, blocked nose. If these symptoms are noticed, it is advised to seek help of a health worker. Meanwhile, you can start giving steam inhalation to the child and apply some soothing balm on the forehead, chest and the nose to alleviate headche and to clear the blocked nose.

For steam inhalation, boil 3-4 mugs of water in a bowl (bhagona). Sit on a chair with the child on your lap. Put the bhagona with steaming water on the floor and cover yourself (with the child) and bhagona in a tent of a bedsheet. Sit there for about 10-15 minutes even if the child cries. Alternatively you can close all doors and windows and then boil water in bhagona on an electric heater in the room itself. Allow the steam to spread in the room for about 30 minutes.

For blocked nose, you can also use home made saline drops. For this, boil water in katori and add about one teaspoonful of common salt. Cool it and saline drops are ready for use. Use one drop in each nostril 4-5 times a day.

Antibiotics and cough syrups are not useful in most of the ARIs and hence should not be used. Infact, these can cause problems.

Keep a watch on child's breathing rate. If the breathing becomes difficult, rapid and there is retraction of the ribs while breathing, it is a warning that you must see a paediatrician at the earliest. It can be pneumonia which will surely require antibiotics for its treatment. Pneumonia can be life threatening.

As in diarrhoea, continue normal feeding of the child during an attack of ARI. Never reduce or stop feeding the child.

Fever

If the child has fever, you should make sure that fever does not go above 102c^{0}. If the fever is high, remove unnecessary clothes from the child's body. You should immediately start therapy with water (called Hydrotherapy). Sponge the child's entire body with wet cloth or leave a wet cloth on the body for 5-10 minutes and reapply by wetting and wringing it again. Keep doing it till fever comes down. Seek help of a health worker.

Other common guidelines for better care of the child (of any age)

- Keep the nails of the child short and clean.
- Wash the head nicely with soap and water to prevent lice or other infestations of the scalp.
- Don't allow the child to become undisciplined. Don't succumb to unreasonable demands of the child. However, do show your affection in abundance through your TLC (Tender Loving Care).
- If the child is otherwise normal but refuses to eat, don't be too anxious. Never force to feed the child. If possible give different food preparations to the child everyday. After all, who does not want variety?
- Contrary to what you might believe, Kajal is of no use to the child's eyes. Avoid it. It will be better if you wash the child's eyes with clean water a few times, every day.

20

Constipation and Its Treatment

Constipation is a condition in which the bowels are evacuated at a longer interval or with difficulty. What the right interval should be, is difficult to generalize since it varies from person to person. Some evacuate their bowels once, others twice a day, while there are others who seek this pleasure only once in 2 or 3 days and yet have sound health.

What Causes Constipation?

Some may have constipation on account of the change of enviornment, or emotional tension, but the normal rhythm returns after a few days, and should not be a source of worry. The most important causes of constipation are a disregard of the call to pass motion and an improper diet. When the rectum is full, it sends signals to the intestines through the central nervous system for their movement and if this is repeatedly ignored it gradually leads to failure of the rectum to signal the urge. The diet should contain a reasonable amount of non absorbable material to form a bulk which acts as a stimulus for the intestinal movements. Highly spicy foodstuffs such as chaat, pickles and hot curries may stimulate the bowel to cause a complete evacuation, but this is followed by inactivity of the intestines and constipation. Similarly, purgatives also stimulate the intestines, to cause their evacuation and this is also followed by constipation. To treat this constipation, again a purgative is needed and this continues in the form of a constipation purgative constipation cycle. Other causes of constipation may be a disease or abnormality of gastrointestinal tract, adverse effects of drugs, drying of the stools (faecal impaction), obstruction of the intestines, and severe illness in which food intake is too small. In case of prolonged constipation in the infants or intermittent constipation with diarrhoea, the physician should be consulted to rule out surgical problems.

What Can Be Done About Constipation?

If you are suffering from constipation, and have been taking purgative, try to stop these gradually. Your system will probably return to normal if you take enough soups, vegctables, fruits etc. However, if you are the worrying type you may take milk laxative only as a temporary measure without making it a habit. Remember, disregarding the call for motion is the worst you can do to your consipation. Do not wait unnecessarily. Rush to the toilet wherever you are, whether at a party or in the kitchen. Your diets should be made up of high roughage foods containing a lot of whole grain cereals, leafy vegetables like spinach, raw carrots and cucumbers, salads, prunes, figs, papaya, water melon and other fresh fruits. Your intestines will soon gain the normal tone. If all these measures fail, you are a candidate for milk purgatives or laxatives. Never take strong purgatives. They are needed only under exceptional circumstances and should be used under the care of a doctor. The purgatives which are commonly used are described here.

Mild Purgatives

Mild purgatives or laxatives are those which promote defecation causing minimum adverse effects. Drugs included in this group are:

Bulk Producing Drugs

Isapgol (at Isabgol), Agar-agar (Agarol), Methyle celluslose.

These drugs absorb water to increase the bulk in the intestines and make the stools soft. The onset of their action is slow, about 12 to 24 hours. They are the safest purgatives for the treatment of chronic constipation. Of the three, isapgol is most commonly used in our country.

Dosage

Isapgol is given preferably with warm milk in a dose of 4 to 5 g once or twice a day. Agar-agar is given in a dose of 4 to 16 g and methyl cellulose in 1 to 6 g in divided doses, for children in the age group of 12-15 years. For younger children the dose should be half.

Adverse Effects

Those agents which are derived from vegetable sources are devoid of toxic effects. Occasionally flatulence may occur, but, this can be relieved by increasing the fluid intake. The chronic use of isapgol may decrease plasma cholesterol by interfering with the absorption of bile acids but it does not cause any harm and may rather do good to an obese patient.

Precaution

Always take plenty of fluids along with these drugs to obtain maximum benefit and to avoid the possibility of intestinal obstruction which has been reported to occur in rare cases.

Stool Softeners

Dioctyle Sodium Sulfosuccinate

This is an effective stool softener for the treatment of constipation in some cases. It is a detergent which absorbs water by reducing the surface tension of fluids in the stools.

Dosage

The daily dose varies from 50 to 500mg depending on the severity of the condition. The action starts after 24 to 48 hours.

Adverse Effects

Adverse effects of this drug are quite rare. It has been reported to interact with mineral oils to increase their absorption.

Precaution

It should not be taken with mineral oils.

Liquid Paraffin (Cremaffin)

This is a traditional remedy for constipation. It is an inert oil which lubricates the intestines and forms a film or coating around the stools to make its passage smooth and comfortable. It softens the stool by preventing the absorption of water into the intestines. It is often recommended to patients of piles, heart attack, and to pregnant women, as well as after surgery on the rectum or abdomen and in cases in which straining to evacuate may be harmful. It is quite popular as it allows the stool to pass through the intestines with a minimum of friction.

Dosage

Liquid paraffin is given in a dose of 15 to 45 ml. Its action starts after 12 to 24 hours.

Adverse Effects

If taken regularly, it may cause deficiency of fat soluble Vitamins such as A, D and K. It may at times leak through the gastrointestinal tract and cause not only annoying but embarrassing situation. Its presence in the rectum inhibits the stimulatory reflexes to the intestines and prevents complete evacuation of bowels. On aspiration, liquid paraffin has also been reported to cause lipoid pneumonia in elderly and weak persons. Although it promotes and facilitates the passage of stools, it delays healing and, therefore, its use is not preferred after surgery for piles.

Precautions

1. It should not be taken regularly as it may cause deficiency of Vitamins A, D and K . This may be very harmful, specially in pregnant women.
2. It should not be taken by very old and weak persons, and young children because of the danger of lipoid pneumonia.
3. It should not be taken during the day time because of chances of its leakage through the rectum.
4. It delays healing, and is not recommended after an operation on piles.

5. It should not be taken along with dioctyls sodium sulfosuccinate, as the latter promotes its absorption from the intestines.

Mild Saline Purgatives

Magnesium Hydroxide

This is a mild laxative which can be used even by pregnant women and children. It absorbs water from the intestines to form the bulk and make the stools soft. Besides purgative action, it counteracts acidity in the stomach.

Dosage

Its usual dose is 2 to 4g its action starts after 2 to 6 hours.

Adverse Effects

It is a mild purgative and does not have any adverse effect except to produce flatulence in some people.

Precautions

1. Take plenty of fluids along with this purgative.
2. Patients with chronic kidney disease who may have difficulty in excreting magnesium should be wary of milk of Magnesia.

Sodium Potassium Tartrate

It is the basic ingredient of commonly used ENO's fruit salt and Seidlitz powder. These also contain tartaric acid and sodium bicarbonate which interact to produce carbondioxide gas, forming an effervescent drink, which resembles gas containing soft drinks . The gas present in the solution distends the stomach and reflexly stimulates movements of the intestines. It also absorbs water from the intestines which assists in forming the bulk and softening the stools.

Dosage

The dose of sodium potassium tartrate for its purgative action is 10g. Its action starts after 3 to 6 hours.

Adverse Effects

Sodium potassium tartrate is a safe purgative and does not cause any adverse effect.

Precautions

It should not be taken by those who are on a sodium restricted diet, e.g. patients of heart failure, hypertension etc, but children are free of all such problems.

Important Note:- The dose should be half of the prescribed dose and keep in touch with your paediatrician.

21

Abdominal Pain and Its Treatment

Abdominal pain, one of the most frequently occurring symptoms, may originate from any organ in the abdomen, like the stomach, intestines, appendix, gall bladder, pancreas and kidneys. There are number of causes for this and therefore, any patient of abdominal pain of recent onset requires early and thorough evaluation for accurate diagnosis. However, the commonest source of abdominal pain in the region of stomach and intestines is the gastrointestinal tract which consists of the stomach and intestines because it deals with outside material, i.e. the food and drink we take. A little overeating may cause distension and indigestion. A spicy meal may lead to an increase in acid secretion and sour eructations. In these conditions some digestives or antacids are taken for relief. Very often flatulence, diarrhoea, dysentery, or an infection may produce spasms of the walls of the intestines causing a gripping type of pain called colic. This is a distressing situation and suitable measures for immediate relief are necessary.

Various house hold remedies like massage, hot water fomentation, churan, ajwain, jaljeera, and sometimes even purgatives are tried, but their success is usually limited. Therefore, the patient takes one of the preparations mentioned as pain killer which provides immediate relief. What is so special about these preparations that they provide such dramatic relief? If you look at the salts of any tablet, you will find that all the preparations contain an antispasmodic (which prevents spasm of the smooth muscle of the intestine). In addition, all these agents contain either a pain reliever or a sedative and some even contain a purgative. Such remedial measures may be effective in mitigating the colicky or intermittent type of pain. However, if it is frequent or of a dull constant nature, the physician must be consulted. Under such circumstances the continued and prolonged use of these drugs instead of improving the condition, may produce serious adverse effects. Since an antispasmodic is the most common ingredient of all these preparations, we will elaborate a little on it.

Antispasmodics

These are atropine or its synthetic substitute (anticholinergic drugs) and are used for relieving the spasm of the muscles of the intestine. The actions of almost all these drugs are more or less the same. There are only slight differences in their potency or duration of action. There may be some adverse effects caused and precautions to be observed with these drugs.

Combinations

After antispasmodics, the next common ingredient in all these preparations is a pain reliever. Some contain a sedative or a tranquillizer as well. Pain relievers may not be of much help unless the spasm is reduced. Undiagnosed pain precludes the use of phenolphthalein, a purgative, even if it is associated with constipation. Phenolphthalein itself aggravates gripping pain being irritant in nature. All these combinations have no greater value than the use of antispasmodics alone apart from increasing the cost and side effects. Some important drugs are Meftolspas, Proxyvon, Colimex, Cyclopam, Buscopan etc. Use only after taking advice from your paediatrician.

22

Stomachache & Gas with Treatment Plan

The distress or stomach ache after eating is actually classified in two ways:

1. ***Distress appearing immediately after eating (postprandial distress):*** symptoms arise half an hour after a meal, such as abdominal bloating, distension, fullness or pressure.
2. ***Intestinal distress:*** Here symptoms usually start half an hour after eating and continue for several hours depending upon person to person. They may involve the stomach, small or large intestines with additional symptoms (to that of postprandial distress) such as abdominal pain and cramps and/or anal flatus.

Excess of gas in stomach and intestines is quite distressing and it is due to the disordered intestinal movements which delays the passages of gases through the bowel. Drugs might provide a symptomatic relief in the following ways:

1. The active ingredients may lower the surface tension of the stomach contents to facilitate the action of digestive juices, which will speed up the digestion and the passage of food contents from the stomach into the intestines.
2. The active ingredients may speed up stomach emptying by changing the stomach's acidity or increasing the contractions of smooth muscles of the stomach or by some other mechanisms.

The commonly available preparations, usually in combination, may contain the following ingredients:

Antiflatulents: Dimethicone (dimethypolysiloxane) and simethicone (a combination of dimethylpolysiloxanes and silica gel) act as antifoaming agent by reducing surface tension. The small mucous covered bubbles of gas (which hold air back) come close to each other, coalesce, and a large bubble is formed which is easily expelled out.

Carminative Oils: Peppermint, cumin, 'azovan' oils, etc. relax the muscles between oesophagus and stomach, increase the gastric secretions and churning in the stomach accelerate the passage of food from stomach.

Antacids: Magnesium trisilicate, light magnesium oxide, sodium carbonate etc. reduce gastric acidity.

Sodium Bicarbonate: It is a household baking soda (mitha-soda) which releases carbon dioxide as it interacts with acid in the stomach. It is useful for relieving distress after meal. Elderly patients above 60 should not consume more than a teaspoonful daily and if one is already on sodium or salt restricted diet, physician approval is necessary. In any case, this should not be used for more than a fortnight, unless a physican directs so.

Charcoal: Activated charcoal and wood charcoal can relieve bloating and other intestinal distress symptoms on account of its absorbent properties. However, it may bind a number of drugs and inactivate them for the same (absorbent) reason. Not more than 10g per day in divided doses would be safe for adults. So, for children the dose should be half.

23

What is Arthritis

There are several different kinds of arthritis, the following are the most common:

Osteoarthritis: Also called degenerative arthritis. Occurs when the cushioning cartilage in a joint breaks down. Commonly affects feet, knees, hips, and fingers. Affects an estimated four crore Indians, mostly 45 years and older. About half of those 65 years and older have this form.

Rheumatoid Arthritis: The body's own immune system attacks the lining, or synovial membrane, of the joints. Joint damage can become severe and deforming. Involves the whole body, and may also cause fatigue, weight loss and anaemia, and affect the lungs, heart and eyes. Affects about 50 lakh Indians, thrice as many women as men.

Gout: Sudden, severe attacks, usually in the big toe, but any joint can be affected. A metabolic disorder in which uric acid builds up in the blood and crystals form in joints and other places. Drugs and attention to diet can control gout. Affects about 30 lakh Indians (almost 80 percent of them men), with the first attack starting between 40 and 50 years of age.

Ankylosing Spondylitis: A chronic disease of the spine that can result in fused vertebrae and rigid spine. Often milder and harder to diagnose in women. Most people with the disease also have a genetic marker known as HLA-B27. Usually affects men between the ages of 16 and 35.

Juvenile Arthritis: The most common form is juvenile rheumatoid arthritis. Its characteristics are different from those seen in adults. Some children recover completely; others remain affected throughout their lives.

Psoriatic Arthritis: The bone and other joint tissues become inflamed, and, like rheumatoid arthritis, it can affect the whole body. Affects about 5 percent of people with psoriasis, a chronic skin disease. Likely to affect fingers or spine. Symptoms are mild in most people but can be quite severe.

Rheumatic Fever: In this fever, fleeting joint pains, malaise, sore throat and affliction of the heart caused by streptococcus infection.

Systemic Lupus Erythematosus: Involves skin, joints, muscles, and sometimes internal organs. Symptoms usually appear in women of childbearing age but can occur in anyone at any age. Also called lupus or SLE, it can be mild or life threatening. Affects nine to ten times as many women as men.

Other Conditions: Arthritis can develop as a result of an infection. For example, bacteria that cause gonorrhea or Lyme disease can cause arthritis. Infectious arthritis can cause serious damage, but usually clears up completely with antibiotics. Tubercular arthritis can affect any joint in the body and will require anti-tubercular medication.

Scleroderma is a systemic disease that involves the skin, but may include problems with blood vessels, joints and internal organs.

Fibromyalgia syndrome is a soft-tissue rheumatism that doesn't lead to joint deformity.

Fibrositis usually occurs mostly in women after childbearing, though it is known to affect teenagers as well. Symptoms worsen with cold and humidity.

Bursitis is a painful inflammation of the bursa—small sacs with fluid that function as shock absorbers between bones, muscles and joints. The area surrounding the joint rather than joint itself is affected.

Are all Joint Pains Signs of Arthritis?

Tennis elbow or epicondylitis of elbow joint is a condition often confused with arthritis. It is caused by overuse of arms, weight lifting, etc. Frozen shoulder or pericapsulitis leads to a loss of motion and causes general pain and tenderness. Same is the case with Achilles Tendinitis, a painful condition of the foot caused by athletic overactivity. These are passing pains and usually disappear after due rest has been afforded to the exerted joint. For example, stiffness in the neck may be of muscular origin and not necessarily arthritis and may actually be a result of sleeping in an awkward position. Many such discomforts disappear after a while, but if pain persists or occurs more frequently arthritis may be suspected. In children, growing pains—which often interfere with children's sleep—may also be mistaken for arthritis, but these require no specific treatment as they shall soon pass.

Warning Signs of Arthritis

According to the US National Arthritis Foundation, the four warning signs to look out for in case of arthritis are:

- persistent pain and stiffness on arising.
- pain, tenderness or swelling in one or more joints.
- recurrence of these symptoms, especially when they involve more than one joint.
- recurrent or persistent pain and stiffness in the neck, lower back, knees and other joints

Diagnosis and Treatment

A common misconception about arthritis is that it is a noncurable disease and the best one can do is manage it by reducing the pain but new research into the mechanism of arthritis and the introduction of path-breaking new drugs is fast changing all that. Arthritis can be successfully combatted and people can get on with their lives without too much hindrance from the disease.

Proper treatment depends on correct diagnosis of the specific disease, and varies with severity and location, as well as from person to person. Diagnosis depends on integrating a host of factors, including the possibility that a person may have two forms of the disease. But treatment need not wait for a final diagnosis because initial treatment options, such as anti-inflammatory drugs and exercise, are similar for many forms of the disease. Treatment should begin early to reduce joint damage.

Generally arthritis is a disease that has days of ups and days of downs. A worsening or reappearance of the disease is called a flare. Remissions bring welcome relief, but can also obscure whether symptoms decreased on their own or due to treatment. This leads to mistaken beliefs in unproven quack cures, and leads to poor drug compliance by the patient, and hence a worsening of the condition in the long run.

24

Arthritis Pain and It's Relief

The pain of arthritis may come from different sources. These may include inflammation of the synovial membrane (tissue that lines the joints), the tendons, or the ligaments; muscle strain; and fatigue. A combination of these factors contributes to the intensity of the pain.

The pain of arthritis varies greatly from person to person, for reasons that doctors do not yet understand completely. Factors that contribute to the pain include swelling within the joint, the amount of heat or redness present, or damage that has occured within the joint. In addition, activities affect pain differently so that some patients dose not feel pain in their joints after first getting out of bed in the morning whereas others develop pain after prolonged use of the joint. Each individual has a different threshold and tolerance for pain, often affected by both physical and emotional factors. These can include depression, anxiety, and even hypersensitivity at the affected sites due to inflammation and .tissue injury. This increased sensitivity appears to affect the amount of pain perceived by the individual.

Measuring Arthritis Pain?

Pain is a private, unique experience that cannot be seen. The most common way to measure pain is for the doctor to ask you, the patient, about your problems. For example, the doctor may ask you to describe the level of pain you feel on a scale of 1 to 10. You may use words like aching, burning, stinging, or throbbing. These words will give the doctor a clearer picture of the pain you are experiencing. Since doctors rely on your description of pain to help guide treatment, you may want to keep a pain diary to record your pain sensations. On a daily basis, you can describe the situations that cause or alter the intensity of your pain, the sensations and severity of your pain, and your reactions to the pain. For example:

"On Sunday night, sharp pains in my knees produced by housework interfered with my sleep; on Monday morning, because of the pain, I had a hard time getting out bed. However, I coped with the pain by taking my medication and applying ice to my knees."

The diary will give the doctor some insight into your pain and may play a critical role in the management of your disease.

What will Happen When You First Visit a Doctor for Your Arthritis Pain?

The doctor will usually do the following:

- Take your medical history and ask questions such as: How long have you had this problem? How intense is the pain? How often does it occur? What causes it to get worse? What causes it to get better?
- Review the medications you are using
- Conduct a physical examination
- Take blood and/or urine samples and request necessary laboratory work
- Ask you to get X-rays taken or undergo other imaging procedures such as a CAT scan (computerized axial tomography) or MRI (magnetic resonance imaging).

Once the doctor has done these things and reviewed the results of any tests or procedures, he or she will discuss the findings with you and design a comprehensive management approach for the pain caused by your osteoarthritis or rheumatoid arthritis.

Who Can Treat Arthritis Pain?

A number of different specialists may be involved in the care of an arthritis patient often a team approach is used. The team may include doctors who treat people with arthritis (rheumatologists), surgeons (orthopaedists), and physical and occupational therapists. Their goal is to treat all aspects of arthritis pain and help you learn to manage your pain. The physician, other health care professionals, and you, the patient, all play an active role in the management of arthritis pain.

How is Arthritis Pain Treated?

There is no single treatment that applies to all people with arthritis, but rather the doctor will develop a management plan designed to minimize your specific pain and improve the function of your joints. A number of treatments can provide short-term pain relief.

Short-Term Relief

- *Medications*: Because people with osteoarthritis have very little inflammation, pain relievers such as acetaminophen (Tylenol) may be effective. Patients with rheumatoid arthritis generally have pain caused by inflammation and often benefit from aspirin or other nonsteroidal antiinflammatory drugs (NSAIDs) such as ibuprofen.
- *Heat and cold*: The decision to use either heat or cold for arthritis pain depends on the type of arthritis and should be discussed with your doctor or physical therapist. Moist heat, such as a warm bath or shower, or dry heat, such as a heating pad, placed on the painful area of the joint for about 15 minutes may relieve the pain. An ice pack (or a bag of frozen vegetables) wrapped in a towel and placed on the sore area for about 15 minutes may help to reduce swelling and stop the pain. If you have poor circulation, do not use cold packs.
- *Joint Protection*: Using a splint or a brace to allow joints to rest and protect them from injury can be helpful. Your physician or physical therapist can make recommendations.
- *Transcutaneous electrical nerve stimulotion (TENS)*: A

small TENS device that directs mild electric pulses to nerve endings that lie beneath the skin in the painful area may relieve some arthritis pain. TENS seems to work by blocking pain messages to the brain and by modifying pain perception.

- *Massage*: In this pain-relief approach, a massage therapist will lightly stroke and/or knead the painful muscle. This may increase blood flow and bring warmth to a stressed area. However, arthritis-stressed joints are very sensitive so the therapist must be very familiar with the problems of the disease.
- *Acupuncture*: This procedure should only be done by a licensed acupuncture therapist. In acupuncture, thin needles are inserted at specific points in the body. Scientists think that this stimulates the release of natural, pain-relieving chemicals produced by the brain or the nervous system.

Osteoarthritis and rheumatoid arthritis are chronic diseases that may last a lifetime. Learning how to manage your pain over the long term is an important factor in controlling the disease and maintaining a good quality of life. Following are some sources of long-term pain relief.

Long-Term Relief

Medications:

Nonsteroidal anti-inflammatory drugs (NSAIDs): These are a class of drugs including aspirin and ibuprofen that are used to reduce pain and inflammation and may be used for both short-term and long-term relief in people with osteoarthritis and rheumatoid arthritis.

Disease-modifying anti-rheumatic drugs (DMARDS): These are drugs used to treat people with rheumatoid arthritis who have not responded to NSAIDs. Some of these include methotrexate, hydroxychloroquine, penicillamine and gold injections. These drugs are thought to influence and correct abnormalities of the immune system responsible for a disease like rheumatoid arthritis. Treatment with these medications requires careful monitoring by the physician to avoid side effects.

Corticosteroids: These are hormones that are very effective in treating arthritis. Corticosteroids can be taken by mouth or given by injection. Prednisotone is the corticosteroid most often given by mouth to reduce the inflammation of rheumatoid arthritis. In both rheumatoid arthritis and osteoarthritis, the doctor also may inject a corticosteroid into the affected joint to stop pain. Because frequent injections may cause damage to the cartilage they should only be done once or twice a year.

- *Weight reduction:* Excess pounds put extra stress on weight-bearing joints such as the knees or hips. Studies have shown that overweight women who lost an average of 11 pounds substantially reduced the development of osteoarthritis in their knees. In addition, if osteoarthritis has already affected one knee, weight reduction will reduce the chance of it occurring in the other knee.
- *Exercise*: Swimming, walking, low-impact aerobic exercise and range-of- motion exercises may reduce joint pain and stiffness. In addition, stretching exercises are helpful. A physical therapist can help plan an exercise program that will give you the most benefit.
- *Surgery*: In select patients with arthritis, surgery may be necessary. The surgeon may perform an operation to remove the synovium (synovectomy) realign the joint (osteotomy). or in advanced cases replace the damaged joint with an artificial one. Total joint replacement has provided not only dramatic relief from pain but also improvement in motion for many people with arthritis.

How Can You Cope with Arthritis Pain?

The long-term goal of pain management is to help you cope with a chronic, often disabling disease. You may be caught in a cycle of pain, depression and stress. To break out of this cycle, you need to be an active participant with the doctor and other health care professionals in managing your pain. This may include physical therapy, cognitive-behavioral therapy, occupational therapy, biofeedback, relaxation techniques (for example, deep breathing and meditation), and family counseling therapy.

Another technique is to substitute distraction for pain. Focus your attention on things that you enjoy. Imagine a peaceful setting and wonderful physical sensations. Thinking about something that is enjoyable can help you relax and become less stressed. Find something that will make you laugh, a cartoon, a funny movie, or even a new joke. Try to put some joy back into your life. Even a small change in your mental image may break the pain cycle and provide relief.

What Research is Being Conducted on Arthritis Pain?

Recent NIAMS studies show that levels of several neuropeptides (compounds produced by cells of the nervous system), such as substance P, are increased in arthritic joints. Substance P is involved in the transmission of pain signals via the nervous system. At the University of Missouri, researchers are studying effects of substance P in the spines of animals with chronic arthritis. Findings from this study may be used to develop specific drugs for chronic pain such as that associated with arthritis.

Researchers are also studying the human knee and analyzing how injury in one joint may affect other joints. In addition, they are analysing the effect of pain and analgesics on gait (walking) and comparing pain and gait before and after surgical treatment of knee osteoarthritis.

25

Medication for Arthritis

The drugs used for treating most types of arthritis are drawn from many categories, but can be thought of in a few broad groups, such as anti-inflammatory drugs and disease-modifying drugs. More than one medication may be required for treating arthritis.

Anti-inflammatory agents generally work by slowing the body's production of prostaglandins, substances that play a role in inflammation. Many have an analgesic, or painkilling effect at low doses. Usually, higher, sustained doses are required to see sufficient anti-inflammatory activity for treating arthritis. The most familiar anti-inflammatory agent is **aspirin**, often a good arthritis treatment.

Like aspirin, **nonsteroidal anti-inflammatory drugs** (NSAIDs) fight pain and inflammation. More than a dozen NSAIDs are available, most by prescription only. Gastrointestinal side effects are common. Like aspirin, NSAIDS also deplete the iron reserves of the body. Take a multivitamin pill with at least 18 mg of iron.

The most potent anti-inflammatory drugs are corticosteroids, synthetic versions of the hormone cortisone, like prednisone and dexamethasone. Usually reserved for short periods of use during intense flares or when other drugs don't control unrelenting disease. Relief can be dramatic, but long-term use causes side effects, such as weight gain, high blood pressure and thinning of bones and skin.

Usually steroids are given orally, but they can also be injected directly into a joint to reduce side effects. Corticosteroids harm the bones by blocking calcium absorption and interfere with vitamin D levels. Consider boosting your calcium intake with a separate calcium supplement.

Disease modifiers slow the disease process in autoimmune diseases such as rheumatoid arthritis or systemic lupus erythematosus. Patients taking these drugs are closely monitored.

It may take weeks or months to learn if a drug works. During that wait, it's important to keep taking other medications such as NSAIDs. A side effect of these drugs is the depletion of folate.

Gold salts have been used to treat rheumatoid arthritis for 60 years, although nobody knows why this treatment works. Penicillamine, methotrexate, and antimalarials such as hydroxychloroquine are also used. Doctors usually reserve other powerful drugs that suppress the immune system for extremely serious disease.

Note: Get off harmful drugs, sleeping pills, tranquilisers, narcotics, painkillers, if you have ben using them for a continued duration. These drugs can become a part of life, and in the long run only worsen your quality of life. It's not that these drugs don't work. They do, but for most people they are needed in ever increasing amounts and end up creating many more problems than they solve.

Tips on Joint Protection

Easing stress on joints is important to avoid further damage. Doctors, physical therapists and occupational therapists recommend canes, walkers or crutches for some people to help lighter the amount of body weight placed on certain joints. They may also help patients learn to use their joints in safer ways. For instance, the whole arm or the side of the body can be used to push a door open instead of the hand. Sliding heavy objects where possible will minimise stress on your weight bearing joints.

You can protect your joints by changing positions frequently to avoid stiffness, taking care to avoid joint positions that may be painful or may put excessive strain on the joints.

Splints may be used to keep joints from becoming permanently bent and stiff. Splints help rest joints, hold proper positions and keep muscles and ligaments around the joints limber. Using a forearm or auxiliary crutch on the opposite side will reduce by more than half the amount of weight borne by the affected joint.

Don't bandage the joints too tightly as this will impair blood circulation.

The Importance of Rest

Too much activity can lead to increased pain and inflammation. Rest helps relieve those effects. On the other hand, too much rest may lead to stiffness and joints that move poorly. The right balance between rest and activity has to be found for each person, and that balance depends on how severe the symptoms are at any given time. More rest and less activity are needed during flares of pain and the opposite is true during periods of improvement.

The basic maxim for those suffering from RA is 'Don't race, pace!' You need to learn how to pace yourself and not try to do everything you can possibly do on the days when you are feeling good. All that it does is make you tired and sore the next day. Remind, yourself to slow down and listen to your disease.

Hot and Cold Treatments

Using heat (hot baths, hot packs, heat lamps etc.) can relax muscles and relieve pain and soreness. And cold (compresses, ice bags etc.) can help numb the affected area and reduce blood circulation to alleviate pain.

Use cold treatments for those times when a joint has been stressed from overuse. When joints become swollen hot or tender, heat is the best solution, cold would make them very painful.

26

What is Osteoarthritis?

Osteoarthritis is destruction of the smooth cartilage covering the ends of the bones. This destruction is similar to the wear and tear of moving machines. It usually starts in the middle age without any specific cause. You may have seen elderly persons walking like a duck, or using a stick to walk. Most of these people suffer from osteoarthritis.

Stages

In early stages there is pain or catch in the knee while :

- getting up from siting position or
- changing position of the knee after a period of rest in one position.

  In later stages, pain is almost constant and becomes worse on exertion. At this stage the pain is relieved by :

- rest;
- pain killer medicines; or
- oil massage.

In advanced stage, walking is difficult and often needs a lot of effort. Going up and down the stairs is especially very difficult. The knee may appear 'swollen' and thigh may appear thin. The shape of the legs changes and the knee bows outwards. At this stage, the gait changes and there may be sideways lurch at every step.

Causes

Common causes of osteoarthritis are:

- Wear-and-tear due to prolonged use of the joint (This is the commonest cause of osteoarthritis);
- Defect in quality of the cartilage such as in a disease called pseudogout;
- Defect in alignment of the articulating surfaces;
- Loose structures inside the joint such as a loose cover of the meniscus;
- Old injury; and
- Previous infection.

Risk groups

Osteoarthritis may run in families. It is more common in obese people and those who use the knee excessively such as for sports, standing for a long time or working for long hours with knee in extreme positions. Osteoarthritis is 10 time more common in females than in the males. People with bowed legs develop osteoarthritis much earlier.

Symptoms

Osteoarthritis of the knee is more common among people above fifty years of age, especially the obese. Most people with osteoarthritis complain of pain and/or creaking sound in the knee.

Many people who believe that knee pain means beginning of old age do not always consult with a doctor. It is important to remember that knee pain can occur at all ages and some causes are curable. Also, there are some diseases which may start as a mild pain but rapidly progress to destroy the knee joint. Early diagnosis and timely management that can prevent the progress of an otherwise progressive disease.

When to consult with a doctor?

You should consult with a doctor, especially orthopedic surgeon if you have:

- Pain or stiffness in one joint only or if one joint is affected more than the other;
- Repeated swelling of the knee with pain;
- Symptoms suggestive of a mechanical fault as sudden clicking, something either moving or loose inside the joint.
- Recent bowing of the legs with pain or the inner side of the knee.
- Walking about within the house is difficult due to pain.

Management

Osteoarthritis is not curable. Once it starts, it remains for rest of the life. However, you can relieve the symptoms and minimise disability with timely treatment. Management of osteoarthritis is through

- non-surgical methods in early stages and
- surgical methods in advanced stages.

Non-Surgical Management

The patient has to do the following for non-surgical management of osteoarthritis.

Patient education. You may start worrying about being crippled because of arthritis. Your doctor will, therefore, give you a very true picture of your condition which will help lessen your fears and anxiety.

Weight reduction. Regular and adequate exercise may be a problem if you have difficulty in walking. You may, however, do cycling or swimming regularly. It is, therefore, important to modify your diet and avoid high calorie foods such as sugar, sweets, rice, potato, oil or ghee.

Avoid the following which put excessive stress on the knee:

- Sitting on the floor, in low chairs, sofa or beds.
- Squatting, sitting cross-legged and using Indian style toilets.
- Exercises in which you have to stand or walk for a long

time.

You may get relief by:

- Doing exercises where you can sit on a chair or stool.
- Doing specific exercises to build up the muscles around the knee for providing support to the 'weak' knee.
- Occasional use of medicines to relieve pain. Paracetamol is a safer medicine.

Surgical Management

Three types of surgeries are recommended for management of osteoarthritis. These include:

- arthroscopy;
- correction of the alignment of the knee; and
- changing the knee joint. None of these surgeries cure osteoarthritis. Your doctor may recommend anyone of these options depending upon the condition of your knee.
- **Arthroscopy.** Your doctor may recommend if you either have.
- mechanical problems such as something stuck or loose inside the joint or
- repeated swelling of the knee joint. Although the relief may be partial or temporary, it is often recommended because it is a safe and 'minor' procedure.

  As mentioned earlier, your doctor can view the inside of the knee directly through an arthroscope and assess the condition of the cartilage covering the bone-ends and the semi-lunar cartilages. Your doctor will also be able to remove (a) any loose or torn pieces of semi-lunar or articular cartilages or
- loose or over-grown tissue lining the knee. The joint will then be washed thoroughly with saline water to completely remove damaged pieces.

- **Correction of alignment of the knee.** Your doctor may suggest a surgery called High Tibial Osteotomy (HTO) to correct the alignment of the knee. This surgery is usually recommended if you have painful osteoarthritis of the knee with bowing of the legs. When your legs are bowed, more body weight passes through the inner side than the outer side of the knee. During the surgery the bone just below the knee is cut and realigned so that the more body weight passes through the outer side of the knee. After this surgery more than seventy percent patients have relief from pain for almost eight to ten years. It is effective for mild to moderate arthritis, and people who are either young or not obese.

  High tibial osteotomy or HTO is a major surgery and requires a plaster cast for a month after the operation. You can however start walking to the toilet with the plaster about one week after the surgery. Your doctor will also recommend physiotherapy for a few weeks after the cast is removed.

- **Changing the knee joint.** This is a relatively new technique in which the damaged ends of the bones of the knee joint are removed and replaced with artificial parts. A cup-like part is fixed on the end of the thigh bone and a plate-like part is fixed on the end of the leg bone with a special glue called bone-cement. The new parts of the knee are smooth and therefore there is no pain during normal movements of the joint. Although this surgery gives instant relief from pain, it is not always effective. You may have to observe several restrictions in movements so that the new joint may last for five to eight years. Also, the artificial knee joint is very expensive. This surgery is usually recommended for people who are not able to walk within the house also.

27

Causes/Symptoms/Treatment & Investigations of Back Pain

Back, having so many parts, makes easy to develop a problem into itself. Anything that puts pressure on the back muscles or nerves can cause pain. Any illness or damage to the spine also can cause pain. The cause of most acute back pain is unknown, but probably is due to minor strains, sprains, and overuse. Emotional stress may add to the pain, especially since it slows the rate of recovery. Other possible causes of back pain include a ruptured intervertebral disc, spinal stenosis, osteoarthritis, anykylosing spondylitis, an injury or accident, rheumatic-related problems or other conditions.

Many of the problems that cause back pain are the result of injury and degeneration of the intervertebral disc. Degeneration is a process where wear and tear causes deterioration. The disc is subjected to different types of stress as we use our backs each day. Bending over results in compression of the disc and may also cause the disc to bulge backwards towards the spinal canal and nerves. The facet joints must also shift to allow the bending to occur. Twisting and bending together is perhaps the greatest stress on the parts of the spine, especially the disc.

Probably, the earliest of changes that occur in the disc are tears in the annulus portion of the intervertebral disc. The annulus is a large round ligament and the tears in the annulus heal the same way as the tears in other ligaments do, that is by scar formation. Scar tissue is not as strong as normal tissue. The repeated cycle of many annular tears healing by scar tissue leads to the disc that finally begins to degenerate.

What happens when the disc begins to degenerate?

As the degeneration of the disc progresses the nucleus pulposus loses some of its water content. It becomes stiff and loses the ability to act as a shock absorber. The process may continue until the disc is collapsed. Bone spurs may form as the body's response to this degeneration. These spurs are thought to be the result of excess motion at the spinal segment. Eventually, bone spurs form around the nerves of the spine as well.

One of the most dramatic injuries to the lumbar spine is the Herniated Disc. In this injury, a tear in the annular ligament allows the nucleus pulposus to squeeze into the spinal canal. If the disc material compresses the nerve root, there is pain, numbness, and weakness in the areas supplied by the nerve. There is a considerable amount of evidence to suggest that it's not only the pressure that plays a part in the symptoms from a herniated disc. The nucleus material that is squeezed out against the nerve seems to set up an inflammatory response in the nerves causing pain.

Symptoms

Low back pain can be divided into two main types:

- Mechanical Type pain
- Compressive Type pain

Mechanical type back pain results from inflammation caused by irritation or injury to the disc, the facet joints the ligaments or the muscles of the back. A common cause of mechanical pain is disc degeneration. A typical muscle strain, or lumbar strain, can also be the cause of mechanical type symptoms. Mechanical type back pain usually starts near the lower spine. Mechanical type pain may also spread to include the buttock and thigh areas. It rarely extends below the knee.

Compressive or neurogenic (meaning nerve related) type pain occurs when the nerve roots that leave the spine are irritated or pinched. A common cause of compressive pain is a herniated disc. The nerves that leave the lower lumbar spine join to form the sciatic nerve. This nerve provides sensation and controls the muscles of the lower leg. Pressure or irritations on the nerve roots of the lumbar spine that come together to form the sciatic nerve can interfere with the normal function of the sciatic nerve. One of the earliest signs of pressure on a nerve root is numbness in the area supplied by the nerve. Pain is commonly felt in the same area, usually extending below the knee to the foot. In cases where there is pressure on a nerve root as it comes out of the spine, it is not unusual for the back itself to be painless. This can be confusing at times since there is no back pain but the problem is located in the lumbar spine. Finally, the muscles that the nerve controls may become weak and the reflexes may disappear. This is because the pressure on the nerve roots interferes with the signals from the brain to the muscles. There is no signal going from the brain to the muscle to tell it to contract.

Spinal stenosis can also cause compressive type pain. In some people, degeneration of the spine can result in a narrowing of the spinal canal—the bony tube where the spinal nerves are located. This causes all of the nerves within the spinal canal to become inflamed, and fail to work properly. One problem that occurs when the tube is too small, is that the nerves can not get enough blood supply to work properly. The nerves may be normal when the body is at rest, but once it is active the nerves need more blood flow to get more oxygen. If the tube is too tight, the blood supply cannot increase. One of the symptoms of this cause is numbness. It may be in one or both the legs. The numbness may become worse with activities. The pain can involve both of the lower extremities. The pain becomes worse on walking and gets better after short periods of rest. Weakness of the muscles of both legs may also occur, and again, this may get worse when activity increases.

In very few cases, a disc herniation can be so big that it fills the entire spinal canal. The immediate pressure on the nerves in the spine may cause paralysis of the muscles that control the bowels and bladder. When the control over the bowels or bladder is lost, it is better to contact the physician immediately. **If the back pain is accompanied by any of the following, the doctor should be consulted:**

- weakness or numbness in one or both legs
- pain going down one leg below the knee
- back pain from a fall or injury
- back pain accompanied by fever
- pain that continues to interrupt sleep after three nights
- back pain that remains after six weeks of home treatment

Diagnosis

To enable the doctor to diagnose the problem correctly the complete history of the back pain should be provided. The doctor may ask a number of questions as listed below:

- What are the symptoms?
- What kinds of aches or pains?
- Where exactly is the pain?
- Where is the pain the most severe?
- When did the pain begin?
- How long it lasts?
- Did something specific cause the back pain, such as an accident or injury?
- What home treatments is undertaken?
- Was there any additional stress when the pain began?
- Is there any other health problems?
- What kind of work does the patient do?
- Types of recreational activities in which the patient participates.

Next, the doctor will make a clinical/physical examination. During the exam, **the doctor may perform any of the following:**

- observe the muscles and joints
- ask to sit and lie down
- ask to move the back in different positions
- observe the most painful area
- check if other areas of the body are tender or painful (such as the kidneys, intestines, or other organs).

If the doctor can identify the likely cause of the back pain, at this point, no further tests will be needed. If the doctor needs more specific information, the following tests may be advised:

X-ray

Studies show that in many cases of routine back pain, X-rays may not initially be necessary. However, the signs and symptoms will determine what type of study should be done. In certain cases, X-rays might indicate that the pain is due to:

- injury in one or more of the back bones
- a tumor in the spine
- a deformity in the spine
- ankylosing spondylitis

CAT Scan (Computerized Axial Tomography)

Only a few people with lower back pain need a CAT scan. If the doctor advises one, a special machine takes an x-ray scan of the area. A computer turns this scan into a three-dimensional view of the back. This helps the doctor see if there is a ruptured disc that can't be seen on regular x-rays; CAT scan also helps in detecting spinal stenosis, tumors and infections of the spinal cord.

MRI (Magnetic Resonance Imaging)

MRI is another way to make very clear pictures of parts of the spine. The MRI does not use X-rays or radioactive dyes. It can provide clearer pictures of soft tissues such as muscles, cartilage, ligaments, tendons and blood vessels in addition to bone structure. To take a MRI picture, the body must be moved very slowly through a tube in the centre of the machine, which contains very powerful magnets. People, who are claustrophobic or whose bodies contain certain kinds of metal objects, may not be able to tolerate the procedure.

The MRI scanner shows the nerves and disc quite clearly. No special dyes or needles are necessary. The MRI scan is, perhaps, too good at showing the anatomic details of the spine. There is a growing body of evidence that suggests that not all abnormalities that show up on the MRI scan are really the cause of the individual patient's problem related to back pain. Abnormalities, such as bulging discs, show up frequently in normal persons who have never had any problem with their back. Hence, it should be kept in mind that a MRI scan is a great test to show the lumbar spine anatomy and it must be correlated carefully with the symptoms so that the findings aren't blown out of proportion.

Types of Back Pain

Back pain may be acute (generally severe, but short-lived), subacute or chronic (long-lasting or occurring often).

Acute Back Pain

- Pain usually lasts from one to seven days.
- Pain may be mild or severe.
- An accident or injury occasionally may cause pain.
- About 80 percent of all back pain are acute.

Subacute Back Pain

- Pain usually lasts from seven days to seven weeks.
- Pain usually is mild and occasionally severe.
- Pain generally is unrelated to other illness.
- About 10 to 20 percent of all back pain are subacute.

Chronic Back Pain

- Pain usually lasts more than three months.
- Pain may be mild or severe.
- Pain may be related to other illness or may have no identifiable cause.
- About 5 to 10 percent of all back pain is chronic.

Structure of Back

The back is held upright by muscles attached to the backbone. Doctors often refer to the backbone as the spine, spinal column, or backbone and find the discs located between each vertebra. These discs are made of cartilage, which is a soft, elastic material, Discs act as cushions, or shock absorbers. Their main job is to protect the joints from wearing out. Most joints contain a slippery substance called synovial fluid that keeps them moving smoothly.

The spinal cord is very important because it transmits electrical signals between the brain and the nerves in the legs, arms, back and other parts of the body. The spinal cord runs through a hole in each vertebra of the upper and middle parts of the backbone, much like a piece of string through a beaded necklace. The space it runs through is called the spinal canal. At times, a message might pain or discomfort. The pain signal is an important one, because it tells that some part of the body needs attention.

A serious injury to the neck or upper back runs the risk of damaging the spinal cord, causing paralysis of the parts of the body below the injury. It should be noted that the spinal cord is not present in the lower part of the backbone. Here the spinal canal contains a sack of nerves, the cauda equina. The backbone, with all its parts, cannot hold itself upright. It needs strong muscles, tendons, and ligaments for support. Muscles help to move or hold the position. Tendons fasten muscles to bones, and ligaments stretch from one bone to another to hold bones together.

Myelogram

During a myelogram, a special liquid dye called contrast medium is injected into the spinal canal then X-rays are taken of the area. The contrast medium can make problem areas show up more clearly on the X-ray. A myelogram may be ordered to detect problems such as spinal stenosis or spinal cord tumors. If surgery is being considered, particularly for a person who has had a serious back injury, many neurosurgeons will require a myelogram beforehand.

Bone Scan

During a bone scan, a very small amount of radioactive liquid is injected into a vein which concentrates in the bones for a short time. A special radioactive detecting machine scans the area of concern to produce a picture. Occasionally bone scans are done to look for damage or tumors in the bones themselves. However, back pain is rarely due to diseases of the bones.

Electrodiagnostic Studies

Electrodiagnostic studies are used to help confirm the presence of nerve compression in the spine. An electrodiagnostic study consists of two tests. One is an electrical test, which is designed to study nerve conduction. In this test the nerve is given an electrical stimulation, and the speed of the impulse is measured. The other test is a needle test called an electromyogram, or EMG. The purpose of this test is to study the muscles for primary disease or for the effect of nerve compression on the muscle. The compression is especially seen in herniated discs or spinal stenosis.

Blood Tests

If the doctor orders blood tests, a laboratory technician will carefully draw a small amount of blood from a vein in the arm, which will be tested in the laboratory. Anyone of the following blood tests may be advised:

- erythrocyte sedimentation rate (sed rate)
- haematocrit and haemoglobin

- white blood cell count
- HLA B-27 test
- chemical profile (SMAC)

Treatment

The treatment of back pain ranges from simple reassurance that nothing is wrong to extremely delicate surgery. Each case is different and treatment must be individualized to meet the circumstances. Treatment falls into two major categories:

- Conservative treatment—which includes exercise, medications, physical therapy and other non-operative therapy.
- Surgical treatment—which includes laminectomy, diskectomy and spinal fusion in selected conditions.

  Treatment for any back condition should involve two goals:

- To relieve the immediate problem
- To reduce the risk-injury

Exercise plays an important role in achieving both of these goals.

More than 85 percent of people with lower back pain improve with minimal treatment in a matter of days. However, if back problems persist, doctors generally prescribe one or more of the following treatments. For some back conditions, the doctor may refer the patient to another specialist such as an orthopedist, rheumatologists; physical or occupational therapist, psychologist, psychiatrist or surgeon.

Rest

The most common treatment doctors recommend for severe back pain is bed rest. Different people require different amounts of rest. Usually, two to three days of staying in bed, except to go to the bathroom, will be enough to ease the back pain. The doctor may be consulted to know if special pillows or devices are necessary to give additional support to the neck, back, or feet.

Heat and Cold

Many people have found that hot and cold treatments help relieve back pain. It is advisable to try both to find out which of the two works best.

Heat relaxes muscles and soothes painful areas. There are many ways to apply heat. Some people like hot showers or baths, while others prefer using heat lamps, heating pads or warm compresses. For the persons having arthritis, heating the muscles first might make it easier to do back exercises. Care should be taken not to fall asleep while using heat.

Cold has a numbing effect. This often helps relieve pain. One of the following methods may be tried for applying cold:

- an ice bag
- a large ice cube used to massage the area
- frozen package of vegetables (peas work best)
- a commercially made cold pack. Be sure not to leave ice on after the skin becomes numb as this could lead to localized frostbite. Persons sensitive to ice or having decreased circulation or sensation should not use cold treatment.

28

Impotency

Why Impotence Shouldn't Be Ignored

The percentage of men suffering from E.D. (Erectile Dysfunction i.e. Impotency) is very high in our society, but for obvious reasons they don't come forward and continue to suffer, despite having strong sexual desires. Imagine what it must be like not being able to have physical relations for 12 to 15 years !

Anyway, more and more research and articles and support groups are required to address this problem, which has assumed massive proportions. After all, the fitness of our apparatus is very necessary for keeping the other half of the society happy!

The Culprit in Your Case

After taking a detailed history with special reference etc. medical problems and lifestyle habits, your andrologist / urologist will administer these tests:

- The Nocturnal Penile Turnescense Test in which a computer is attached to the penis at night, to check for erection.
- Intra Penile Injections increase the blood flow to the penis and result in an erection which is observed and rate.
- A Penile Ultra Sound Colour Doppler visualizes the blood vessels in the penis.

Mind or Matter?

It is Psychological if

- you wake up with an early morning or middle-of-the-night erection.
- you have had satisfactory interactive intercourse.
- you masturbate perfectly well.
- your problem occurred suddenly.

It is Physical if

- your erection is feeble and does not strengthen even while you sleep, wake up in the morning, or masturbate.
- you fail again and again.
- the onset is gradual.

Irksome Illnesses

By far the most common illnesses that cause impotence is diabetes; over half of all older diabetics have or will have erectile difficulties; 20% of hypertensive can suffer, too.

Other culprits are high cholesterol, spinal injury, pelvic surgery, excessive drinking and smoking which damage the blood vessels.

Incidentally the latest research shows that if you suffer from vascular erectile dysfunction, It is wise to have a cardiac check up, because a link has been established between furred arteries of the penis and faculty arteries of the heart.

With added medical awareness, prescribed drugs such as antihistamines and antidepressants are being held responsible for only 10% of the cases.

Hormone imbalances are even rarer, account for a more 1 %.

Something For Everyone

Treatments for impotence are available for every age, condition, need, preference or social situation.

Homeopathic Medicines

Lycopodium

It is the most famous homeopathic medicine. Famous serologist of U.S.A. Dr. Nash M.D. says that if taken in proper dose this drug not only makes youth robust filled with abundant semen, it even revitalize the sexual potency of the old persons. The effect of the medicine is not temporary but permanent one, hence it should be administered in fixed intervals of time. This medicine is available in various potencies, from 200 to 10000 or even of one lakh potency. The higher the potency the better would be the results. But it is advisable that these medicines should be taken after proper medical advice. Or else they create quite serious complications. This medicine is especially recommended for those strayed youth who ruin their sexual potency by constant use of their male organ. In fact his medicine should be taken by increasing its potency gradually. The medicine of 200 potency should be given on empty stomach to the patient and the next dose of higher potency after one full week. The same way the potency should be increased from 1000 to the dose of the desired potency when the affliction is cured.

Phosphoric Acid

It is also a wonder homoeopathic drug to cure sexual weakness. The constant malpractice result in the patient's face becoming pale and sallow, eyes sunken in the sockets and constant complaints of pain in the waist. The afflicted person's semen also becomes very thin and often passes out with urine while passing stool. This medicine is also good for those patients afflicted with diabetes. It not only enhances the physical power of the patient but makes him very strong mentally also. This medicine is to be administered mixed with three to five drops of mother tincture diluted with 25 to 30 gms. of water. Ask the patient to have the medicine before taking his meal. Phosphoric acid is a powerful drug and should not be administered on empty stomach.

Avenasativa

The cautious use of this celebrated medicine administered mixed with five to six drops of mother tincture is an unfailing remedy for all the sexual weakness. A timid listless boy turns into a robust man by the use of this medicine. It not only strengthens the user's body but increases the efficiency of his mental faculties.

Caution

All these medicines are to be taken after proper medical advice. Don't rush to take them without consulting some good homoeopathic physician. Other good remedies are caladium, conium, staphysagria, and selenium.

29

Dysmenorrhoea (Menstrual Cramps)

Finding the Homeopathic Medicine

- If there is heavy, bright red bleeding, gushing and throbbing pain, look first at Belladonna.
- If the pain is lessened by heat and pressure, think first of Magnesia phosphorica, then of Colocynthis.
- For pain is very intense and the woman is terribly angry and inconsolable, look at Chamomilla.
- If the woman feels better when drawing her knees up to her chest, give Colocynthis.
- If the pain began after anger, think of Nux vomica, Colocynthis, and Belladonna.
- If the pain came on after too much alcohol or rich food, give Nux vomica.

Self Care and Home Remedies

- Alternating hot and cold sitz baths: soak in tub of moderately hot water for five minutes, then in a tub of cold water up to the navel with knees bent for one minute. Alternate two to three times.
- Walking stretching and other physical exercise can sometimes help.
- For muscle cramps, Calcium and Magnesium can help.
- Take Viburnum tincture: one half teaspoon every hour, up to six doses. The dosage for capsules depends on the

specific product.

- A heating pad is often helpful.
- Castor oil packed to the abdomen with a heating pad can sometimes relieve discomfort.
- Avoid caffeine and salt premenstrually.

30

Leucorrhoea

It is generally called a 'white discharge' or simply 'the whites'. In reality, leucorrhoea is a state where there is catarrhal discharge from the Vagina's mucous membranes. This is the most agonising disorder for the females and distorts their health. It may last a life-time or prolong for sometime and then abate or may appear as and when her health is in poor state.

Leucorrheal Flow

- The discharge is often white, like white portion of an, egg or milk-colour, or else it may be off white, yellow, reddish or pinkish, green or light blue, but in most of the cases, it is odourless and white.
- Flow may stiffen the linen or simply leave back a trace of white powder or scales.
- It may excoriate vulva and thighs and the itching caused is sometime too intense and so much that blood oozes out from the site itched.
- Consistency of discharge varies-from water to consistency of cream, milk, viscous fluid or even albuminous.
- In most cases discharge emanates from the uterine cavity or vagina. In catarrhal or idiopathic variety of leucorrhea, the discharge is in mild and liquid form but does not excoriate or irritale the parts. But, when it is dependant inflammation organic lesions of uterus or its appendages the discharged becomes fetid, corrogive, acrid, browish or green.

- The discharge from the uterus is often from uterine cavity, more albuminous, thick, viscid, flocculant, and has an allkaline reaction, whereas vaginal discharge is always acidic, thin, white, creamy and milky.
- Leucorrhoeal discharge is more profuse and copious at the time of menses than at any other time but in some ladies, it continuously goes on, though quantity of discharge varies.

Effects of Leucorrhoea

- If the discharge is copious and continues for a much longer period, there could be heaviness in the epigastriurn and pain. There is also capricious hunger, nausea and vomiting, fainting spells, desire for those things which have no relation to the malady; digestion is difficult and slow; vertigo, headache; slow motion and general lathargy, pain particularly in shoulderblades and generally in all the limbs; face is pale, livid, skin is discoloured and dull.
- When the leucorrhoeal discharge continues for a fairly long period, the patient feels exhausted even on any attempt to slight exertion. She grows weak and then, palpitation and breathlessness, dull and vacant looks, margin of eyes surrounded by black rings, all intellectual faculties are weakened, face is bloated.

Causes of Leucorrhoea

- Affects mostly nervous, lymphatic, feeble, cachetic ladies who have fair complexion, pale skin and soft skin.
- No age is immune from its attack—it can occur anytime between 15-45, though even children at the fairly much yonger age (say 8-10) have been the sufferers.
- There is hardly any endemic leucorrhoea, though undoubtedly some regional foods are deficient in certain elements whic trigger episode of leucorrhoea.
- Depression, self mortification, brooding, chagrin, sudden shocking news or death, loss etc.

- Eating oysters, crabs, fish, acid fruits, hard water, beer, cider, too much use of tea, coffee, purgatives.
- Self-vice or onanism, too much indulgence in sex act, nymphomania, presence of foreign bodies within vagina (like pessaries, sponges etc.)
- Menstrual irregularitis, vaginitis, uterine displacements, pregnancy, miscarriage, worms in intestines, confinement, easy-going life style, pulmonary pthisis, chronic constipation.
- Piles, diarrhoea, suppression of sweat, milky secretion, bronchial expectoration, vomiting, cold in the head.
- Cancers and ulcerations, local inflammations engorgement of cervix (neck of the uterus).
- Presence of gonorrhoea, resulting in inflammation, chancres, other growths.

Leucorrhoea of recent origin is not, at all, difficult to cure but, when in chronic form, treatment is not only difficult but much tedious also, as one has to cure not only leucorrhoea but also other concomittant symptons. Complications accompanying this disease are most difficult to cure than the main disease itself.

31

Causes and Complications of Obsesity

"It is a condition in which excess fat accumulates in the body, mostly in the subcutaneous tissues. Obesity is usually considered when a person is 20 % above the recommended weight for his / her height and build." and how obesity is caused, "The accumulation of fat is caused by the consumption of more food than is required for producing enough energy for daily activities." and also that "obesity is the most common nutritional disorder of recent years."

Obesity is the most common nutritional disorder in affluent societies. Its significance requires constant emphasis because it is associated with increased mortality, predisposes to the development of important diseases and diminishes the efficiency and happiness of those affected" and also that "obesity may be defined as a condition in which there is an excessive amount of body fat. This simple definition gives rise to two questions : how can body fat be measured and what is excessive ?"

Conclusions:

1. It (obesity) is a condition of excessive fat accumulation in the body.
2. Fat accumulates in the subcutaneous tissues.
3. A person is obese when he / she weighs 20% above the recommended weight (in relation to his / her height and build).

4. Fat accumulation is caused by excessive intake of food as compared to depleted energy expenses.
5. It (obesity) is a most common nutritional disorder more particularly of the elite class.
6. It is associated with increased mortality (higher death rate).
7. It is a causative of many killer and non-killer disorders.

Obesity, in itself, is not a disease but it is a most potent factor in causing diseases which are manageable and controllable, provided the obese person adheres to recommended course of dietary regimen, regular and sustainable physical activity, coupled with requisite energy expansion.

Complications triggered by body of over weight

1. Diabetes Mellitus
2. High Blood Pressure
3 Arterio-sclerosis
4. Respiratory problems like breathlessness (dyspnoea) or effort-onset dyspnoea.
5. Early exhaustion and panting even on minimal movement / exertion / effort.
6. Pains and aches in bones, bone-joints, muscles, paving the way for arthritis, osteoarthritis, gout, rheumatism, arthritis deformans, rheumatoid arthritis etc.
7. Acidity, flatulence, colic, constipation or diarrhoea, and other digestion-related disorders.

If we closely look at the information provided above, it is quite easy to conclude that:

(i) Diet
(ii) Exercise or Activity

Are the foremost causatives of overweight but there are still glaring instances when:

- Someone doesn't eat much but is still on the obese side.
- A person may eat more, as a matter of habit, but may not

be obese and lead an active life.

- A frail and scarcely built person also may have physical problems, in spite of good food and physical activity.
- Those who eat more are not necessarily overweight and those who eat far less till gain weight.

All the said variable situations do point to one factor, that is eating does not seem to have much relation to overweight but, conversely, it also cannot be denied, on the basis of statistics available, that excessive and frequent intake of food is still considered to be the biggest monster in causing obesity.

Causes of Overweight

This aspect is a ticklish problem, like a crossword puzzle, due to many hypothesis and variant views expressed in this regard. But, there are still some factors over which most of dieticians and doctors agree. Following factors may contribute to excess body fat, leading to overweight and resultant obesity:

1. Overeating
2. Lack of physical activity
3. Excessive intake of carbohydrates and fats
4. Age factor
5. Endocrine glands malfunctioning
6. Heredity

Overeating and Food

Food is meant to generate energy in the body so as to enable each and every body organ to discharge its individual functions. About eating we must not overlook or ignore undernoted points :-

(i) Eat only when one is real hungry.

(ii) Eat daily at a fix time.

(iii) Diet should include cereals, pulses, seasonal green and leafy vegetables, fruits, fats (in moderate quantity), milk and milk products etc. In a way daily diet should be a balanced and nutritious diet, consisting of above mentioned food items which should also be rich in minerals and vitamins.

(iv) Avoid foods that cause constipation, loose motions, acidity, flatulence, abdominal colic, sour and acidic eructations, belching etc.

(v) Avoid foods which are fried and rich in condiments.

(vi) Use only unsaturated vegetable oils like, soyabean, sunflower, palm, cotton seed oil etc. which reduce cholesterol level.

(vii) Avoid using clarified butter, oil, coconut oil, lard, olive oils and butter which raise cholesterol level, thus causing high blood pressure, cardiac disorders, obesity, joint pains and immobility.

(viii) Dietary fibre, obtained from whole grains, vegetables, and fruits should be used in sufficient quantity. Diet, rich in fibre content, is capable of reducing food intake, as it imparts a sense of satiation to the body.

Gluttons must resist the temptation of eating every time. It disturbs the digestive systems and denies rest to digestive organs and other body organs. Labourers, masons, carpenters, persons employed in construction work, mechanics who have to manually operate heavy machinery and equipment, farmers, children in growth-stage, pregnant ladies, lactating mother. Ladies approaching menopause have to ingest more food than those persons who have to work in an office, shopkeepers, shop employees. If food is not taken in proportion to the expended energy, such a category of persons are liable to get weak but, if persons doing light work also eat heavily, they will be generating more energy which is actually not required.

Operating is also the result of those who sit idle as they have no other activity to perform. Such persons revel in excessive eating as if overeating is the be-all and end-all of their life. When energy is generated through overeating, but no activity is performed to expend the generated energy, it will simply in overweight. For the obese persons overeating is a luxury and a pastime, but for the more hard working persons, sufficient food, to compensate for the energy loss suffered, is a prime necessity.

Calorie Factor

The energy that we derive from diet / food is measured as 'Calorie' which, in fact, is an energy measuring unit and the calories burnt (during the course of physical exercise and exertion). Number of calories burnt / expended, amount of labour put in to a discharge one's work in relation to age, sex, climate. A child, during the growth stage and also during playing games, an old person leading a sedentary life style, a person working in an office, a manual labourer, a stone-cutter, tree-feller, a pregnant woman, during and after pregnancy, a hospitalised patient will require different percentage of calories. Simple rule is : the more energy one spends, the higher calories he would require. When we talk of calorie, total calories required by a person during duration of 24 hours will be reckoned by total calories, obtained from various sources of nutrition. Two persons of the same height, age and workload, would require, different amount of calories because metabolism of each person differs. Every one is a law unto himself, when above criteria are taken into consideration. Two main groups, viz. vegetarians and non-vegetarians, have to work out food items which, when combined, give total calories required by a person. There is another class which adheres to both the said types of food categories.

As already indicated, a balanced diet must be a unified entity, consisting of cereals, green vegetables, fibre, fruits, milk and its various products, meats etc. so that the dietary intake presents a homogenous combination of essential carbohydrates, proteins, fats, minerals, vitamins etc. It is a myth that costly foods give better nutritious values than the cheaper ones but, luckily, the facts is the other way round. So, when working out on your food and diet, you should be more conscious of the nutritional factor than the cost factor. Main purpose is and should be to meet calorie requirement of the body than the money spent therefore.

Dietary Fibre

Fibre is the material which makes the cell walls in the plants and is the indigestible portion thereof. It is neither absorbed by the body nor can it be broken down by the enzymes. In earlier days, it was considered to be a useless matter and was not accorded and therapeutic usage and utility. But, the actual position is that if fibre is discarded and eliminated from our diet, water cannot hold on to the body, thus causing dryness of faeces which results in constipation. It also helps in free movement of intestines and almost rules out inflammation and dryness of intestines, alongwith accumulation of toxi subsistence therein.

Fibre is found in two major kinds: Soluble and insoluble. Certain vegetables and grain cereals have more insoluble fibre. Barley, oats, legumes and fruits contain more soluble fibre. The former (insoluble fibre) aids in removing costiveness and improves digestion, whereas the latter (soluble fibre) helps to lower the serum cholesterol but raises proportion of the good cholesterol, HDL (High Density Lipoprotiens).

In support of our opinion we would like to add Dr. Bukite's expert opinion. "Diets, high in fibre and low in fat, yield soft, moist and plentiful stools, eliminate the need for straining, and are of great help in preventing and treating not only constipation, but (also) haemorrhoids and varicose veins." High fibre diets are required to be chewed for a longer time and, more time is spent in chewing, the less amount of food intake would ensue. It will also give satisfaction and sweetish taste, by constant mixing of saliva, resulting in quick and proper digestion. Since fibres lower insulin levels and thus, lowered insulin secretion will not stimulate appetite. The general rule, in this regard, is that the more the insulin, the more the appetite, and more the appetite, the more intake of food—the last one being the reason for obesity, diabetes and other disorders. So, one can easily infer and deduce that high fibre foods would reduce dietary intake. High soluble fibre foods stay for longer time in the stomach and, thus, there is a feeling of satiated fullness.

Above reasons would suffice to justify an intake of high fibre foods in greater quantity so as to shed weight and stay trim.

"Fibre discourages us from eating more than we (actually) need. Fibre is unique in that it satiates but does not supply calories." If you take juice of two apples and eat two apples, you will feel that, after taking juice, you are again ready to eat, but not so after eating apples and the biggest surprise is that difference is only of 3 gms of fibre per 100 gms of juice / raw apples.

Fibre is a bulking agent. It helps information of stool and renders it bulkier. For smooth passage of stools, it is essential that it should be soft, compact, bulky and smooth so that it passes through the rectum without pain, exertion or strain.

Highly fat-rich foods / diets should be replaced by high fibre diets, especially by heart and cancer patients (in case they are not bed - ridden or inactive). Dr. Burkitt opines thus. "A high fibre diet tends to lower the blood pressure of hypertensive patients", "Research has shown that pectin, the fibre found in the skin of fruits, vegetables and sunflower seeds, will lower blood cholesterol levels." (Quoted respectively from *British Med. Journal* and *American Journal of Clinical Nutrition).*

Lack of Physical Activity

Labourers and others, performing vigorous activity need not undertake any extra exercise, as the jobs done by them suffice to expend the calories. The main problem lies with easy chaired persons, office workers, shop girls / boys who have to stand for long hours, elite people, sedentary and inactive housewives, children who do not play any game or exercise.

Advantages of Physical activity

1. Helps to keep digestive system in functional condition.
2. Tones up circulation of blood.
3. Maintains flexibility of body.
4. Improves cardiac rhythm and output.

5. Helps in normal respiration.
6. Energies blood vessels and doesn't allow cholesterol deposit therein.
7. Improves skin condition, improves complexion, opens up pores of the skin and lets out toxins through sweating.
8. Removes constipation and improves peristaltic action of intestines, rectum and anus.
9. Doesn't allow muscles and joints to become rigid.
10. Dispels pains and aches in body organs, by feeding them with fresh body supply.
11. Tones up nervous system.
12. Doesn't allow extra fat to accumulate.

Ways to Maintain Physical Activity

- Daily morning walk and stroll after taking dinner.
- Attending to calls of nature, taking bath, maintaining a high standard of personal hygiene.
- Performing Pranayama and Yogasanas.
- Aerobic exercise or Push-up exercises.
- Maintaining regularity in daily chores and doing job-related work.
- Not sticking to one posture for longer period.
- Cycling, running, gymnastic exercises.
- Playing games, like badminton, tennis, football, hockey, cricket, kho-kho, kabaddi, swimming, table tennis, jumping, skipping etc.

Remember, playing cards, chess, carrom board, video games, watching TV / Movies, reading newspapers, gossiping, sitting idle for hours together, doing desk-work etc. do not form part of physical activity. In fact these help to add weight to body, hence these are impediments to healthy living and are not only injurious to health but an open invitation to host of diseases which could have been averted, if a person starts doing anyone of the exercise patterns described above.

Hazards of Inactivity

(i) Disturbed digestion.

(ii) Cardiac or Pulmonary dyspnoea.

(iii) Blood Pressure, headache, aching in eyes, and tiredness thereof.

(iv) Rough skin with foul-smelling perspiration or even total / partial absence of perspiration.

(v) Pain and stiffness in neck, shoulders, arms, hands, upper and lower back, hip-joint, knees, legs and feet.

(vi) Even minimal efforts brings on fatigue, soreness, lethargy and there is total dis-inclination even to moderate activity.

(vii) General weakness, rundown condition, apathy, indifference, agitated behaviour, easy proneness to infection.

(viii) Low physical resistance and body's defence mechanism is thrown to shambles.

(ix) Nerves, muscles and bones cry for nutritional supplementation.

Who Should Perform Exercises

Any healthy person of any age should not hesitate to perform anyone of the exercise related activities which must commensurate with amount of food intake and nature of job. Sports persons and athletes have been seen to be quite regular in taking exercise daily. Housewives who perform all or most of the domestic chores need not take to any extra physical activity since dusting, cleaning of floor, washing clothes, making purchases from the market are sufficient activities for them to keep fit and healthy.

Children and young persons should play outdoor games and sports to keep fit and expend the energy and also that their diet also must be such as to meet requirements at the growth stage. They should resist from playing indoor games (except table tennis, if played in a room or courtyard). Moreover they must develop the habit of doing their own work themselves, instead of depending on their family members or servants.

For old and aged persons early morning walk and simple stroll after dinner will suffice to meet their demands on physical activity, provided they do not suffer from any incapacitating disorder. If they are unable to resort to walking, they should simply perform Pranayama and other breathing exercises and also light physical exercises which do not interfere with their physical status / disability. But they must avoid any activity where jerks or falls are feared or anticipated. Even bathing is a good exercise for them, but heart patients must consult their doctors before taking to any activity.

You may or may not derive desired results by doing any physical activity or advantages may be noticed quite late, if done properly but, an exercise done wrongly is bound to harm the body. Adventurous games like trekking, hill climbing, swimming, some aerobic exercises should be done under guidance of the concerned coach.

Persons who should Avoid Physical Activity

Persons who suffer from acute attack of asthma, severe and excruciating headache, backache, stiff and totally immobile joints, in febrile conditions, cancer of any aetiology, after any operation, during the course of travelling, mental agitation, pregnant ladies, debilitated and incapacitated old persons, weak and undernourished children / young persons, stomach ulcers, cirrhosis and cancer of liver, heavy drunkards, chain smokers, drug addicts, traumatic cases should not perform any physical activity or exercise without advice of the attending doctor. If they take to any physical activity of their own, they are simply inviting a calamity for themselves and a problem for other house inmates.

Similarly, no exercise should be performed immediately after return from daily work, in extreme cold, heat and moist weather and when it is raining. Patients to asthma and other respiratory disorders are warned not to venture in performing any physical exercise / vigorous activity when there is an acute attack. Further, when the body is drenched with preparations, when breathlessness sets in, when visibility is poor, weather conditions are not congenial, when stomach is full, or after prolonged fasting. These unfavourable conditions apply to all age groups and both the sexes.

Excessive Intake of Fats

Fat is an essential part of our diet and it is height of imprudent discretion to totally eliminate fats from daily diet. For a normal diet daily consumption of 25 gms is a usual standard requirement. Only saturated fats cause havoc in the form of raised serum cholesterol level which results in raised blood pressure, arteriosclerosis, coronary heart disease, excessive fat accumulation in the body which is the prime factor in obesity and overweight.

Carbohydrates are obtained from sugar, rice, wheat, jaggery, fruits and some vegetables and energy to body is provided by them. It is a fact that heat generated by fats is almost double the amount of energy generated by carbohydrates. Fats are also essential for mobility of joints. But, in order to digest the fats, rigorous and hard activity is required. Excessive ingestion of fats and carbohydrates is responsible for adiposity (obesity).

Fats discharge following functions viz. :

1. To provide protection to body organs.
2. To store energy in the body.
3. To promote growth of body organs by providing necessary fats and
4. To retain the generated head within the body.

Excessive fat consumption finds its way through stools as it is not absorbed within the body. Fat and overweight persons have immense capacity to cat and also digest, and this is the reason as to why fat accumulates in their bodies. It is a fashion in elite and well to do families to eat fat-rich friend foods which are overloaded with carbohydrates also.

There are 3 types of fats viz :

(i) Saturated Fats—These are (saturated) fatty acids that raise serum cholesterol level.

(ii) Polyunsaturated Fats—These fats do not raise serum cholesterol levels.

(iii) Monosaturated Fats—These fats bring down serum cholesterol level and are also known to raise HDL.

Following comparative table will clearly show presence of above mentioned types of fats.

Note: Mark - denotes Fat Contents not known.

30 % of total calorie requirement should be met through unsaturated fatty acids and not from saturated ones. It is necessary that total intake of unsaturated fats should be equally spread over and divided within a period of 24 hours so that there is a regular supply of such fats to all the body organs and production of energy is also uniform. In any case a normal person may consume 25-30 gms of fats daily in divided ones. The said quantity may be raised in the case of persons doing strenuous manual work, irrespective of sex and age.

Carbohydrates

Optimum energy is generated by carbohydrates in the body. Crystal sugar, jaggery, barley, gram, corn/maize, rice, sugars obtained from vegetables (like beets, sweet potato etc), fruits like grapes, mangoes, cherry, apricot, dates, raisins, coconut (fresh), currants, apples, oranges, sweet lime etc. Carbohydrates obtained from fruits metabolise quickly as compared to the ones generated by grain cereals. In diabetes carbohydrates, in excessive quantity, are prohibited but must not be totally eliminated from daily diet. Milk, cheese, yeast, honey have also carbohydrates whereas cow's / goat's milk, Yogurt have low calorie carbohydrates. In obesity, role of carbohydrates cannot be denied.

If a person consumes too much of carbohydrates and fat containing food, his weight is bound to increase. If an ailing and bed-ridden patient resorts to too much intake of carbohydrates, but is not in a position to take to physical activity, he is bound to gain weight and may even become a diabetic or, at least, get prone to the risk of diabetes.

Malfunctioning of Endocrine Glands

"An endocrine influence on body fat is seen both in normal physiological situations and in pathological states. The normal content of young adult woman is twice that of youngman, and pregnancy is characterised by an increase in body weight. Obesity in woman commonly begins at puberty, during pregnancy or at the menopause. Obesity frequently, but not invariably, accompanies hypothyroidism, hypogonadism, hypopituitarism and cushing's syndrome. However, the overwhelming majority of obese patients show no clinical evidence of an endocrinc disorder. Plasma insulin and cortisol are commonly raised and growth hormone reduced in obese subjects, but these changes probably result from, rather than cause, the obesity, since they disappear when weight is lost.

Hypothyroidism is not a decided factor in causing obesity, though, in some obese patients it is also the cause. Deficiency of this hormone can be effectively met with administration of tablets of thyroxine (available in 25, 50, 100 mg tablets) but strictly under medical advice and supervision.

Age Factor

Obesity is generally prevalent in middle age, but it could occur at any stage of life. Weight gain at pregnancy, after delivery, at the time of or after menopause, is quite common. But if a child or adolescent becomes obese at these stages, he will most likely remain an obese in adult life also. After delivery most ladies, irrespective of age, have heavier buttocks, thick thighs, pendulous abdomen and large-sized breast, and all these changes help them towards obesity but, during course of time, most of them regain their former weight, if they continue with recommended exercises. Persons suffering from gout and other disabilities put on extra weight due to lack or absence of physical activity—here age is no bar. If a crippling disability afflicts a person, he can gain weight at any stage of life.

Heredity

It is not necessary that obese parents will necessarily have obese children. Even twin babies do not have an identical weight.

Percentage of Various types of Fat found in oils

S.No.	*Fats oils*	*Saturated Fatty Acids*	*Mono unsaturated Fatty Acids*	*Poly unsaturated Fatty Acids*
1.	Butter oil	65	37	4
2.	Coconut oil	91	6	3
3.	Corn oil	13	26	61
4.	Cotton seed oil	28	19	53
5.	Lard	43	45	12
6.	Olive oil	53	37	10
7.	Peanut oil	18	49	33
8.	Sunflower oil	11	22	67
9.	Soyabean oil	16	24	60
10.	Sesame oil	16	41	43
11.	Mustard Oil	-	-	25
12.	Rice Bran	-	-	35
13.	Vanasapati	-	-	6

Similarly, slim and trim parents also have obese children and vice versa. But genetic and environmental factors do play an important role, as effects of environment, in certain regions of our country, daily use of carbohydrates and fats is customary and inmates of such areas are seen to be generally obese. There is no denying fact that food habits play a significant role in pushing up weight. During the last 25 years, there has been a progressive increase in the percentage of obese and overweight people. Children of obese parents have high risk factor in inheriting obesity from their parents but, even then, exceptions arc still many.

Sundry Causes of Obesity

Socio-Economic Factors

Obesity is more common in lower socioeconomic groups of affluent countries, but in developing countries obesity is more common in the prosperous elite class. Occupations of cooks and barmen are more prone to obesity while front desk receptionists, fashion designers, models, air hostesses, airline pilots, society girls have to keep slim and trim figures. Similarly, film actors and actress, extras, society girls, call girls, prostitutes have also to keep themselves slim to ensure themselves a longer stay in their respective professions.

In some societies fat women and men earn a place of status and are respected but, in others, fat people are neither respected nor considered attractive.

Drugs

Use of oral contraceptives, steroids, insulin and phenothiazines is generally followed by weight gain due to stimulation of appetite. When indoor patients are kept on medication for longer period, their weight normally does not increase but, after their return to homes, they start to take prescribed medicines—it is as if a convict has been released from a jail and, in a spirit of vengeance, he throws all the earlier imposed restrictions to winds and feels free to eat any type of food.

Alcohol

Alcohol as such, may not be a precipitating factor in causing rise in body-weight but drunkards usually follow drinks with meat / fish, fried and heavily spiced vegetables, rice or bread, extra fats in the form of butter, clarified butter, dry fruits. Heavy meals is not uncommon in drunkards as, when in a drunken state, they cannot distinguish between good or bad food, which food is harmful and what quantity is actually needed. Operating is a consequence of drinking, followed by rise in body weight, acidity, vomiting, sour and acidic eructations, flatulence, abdominal colic etc.

Fasting

Fasting is a cleansing process which helps to divest the body from harmful toxins and also affords well deserved rest and holiday from diet consumption, even though for a specific period only. It is held that no food should be taken during fasting but some people do take ice-creams, cold drinks, sweetmeats, sweets, chocolates, so that 'they don't feel weak'. Ladies, though not all, utilise fasting as an effective means to satiate their hunger for abundant rich diet, and also do not hesitate to ingest even the prohibited foods. All these habits lead one to obesity.

Tendency to obesity

In certain families obesity can be commonly seen and the reasons for putting on extra weight are too many to count. Despite best efforts, there is no shedding of weight. Here genetic factor could be the possible factor in adding to body weight. It is not that excessive food intake is generally the contributory cause, apart from sedentary life style. Obese parents can, at least, educate, motivate and guide their siblings about hazards of overweight. It would be still better, if parents and elderly people invite the young ones to join them in weight reducing exercises.

32

Naturopathy—To Reduce Weight

According to this therapy, food, wrong (food) eating habits, eating every time not giving rest to digestive organs, overloading stomach with frequent and unwanted food items, constipation, lack or absence of sweating, interrupted urinary flow, vitiation of three humours, improper and inadequate rest or dietary habits, use of health damaging items like alcohol, tobacco, tea, coffee, intoxicants and drugs, excessive use of spicy, fatty, condiments foods which have bulk or roughage. Unbalanced and nutritionless food etc. are the major causes of various types of disorders, out of which obesity and its offshoot disorders form major diseases we normally suffer from.

Naturopathy aims at excretion of toxins and waste matters from our body through fasting, enema, by inducing perspiration, regulating bowels and urinary flow. Even Ayurveda subscribes to all the said methods when it apologises efficacy of fasting, purging, catharsis, purification (shodhan), sweating (swedana) etc. All such devices are supplementary to the leading curative method, by whichever name we may call it.

Since our main subject is obesity, I will confine myself only to the methods which help to purge the body, normalises breathing and circulatory and cardiac efficiency, promotes and facilitates free flow of urine, expulsion of facial matter (stools), induce sweating, keep up mobility of limbs and, above, all general maintenance of health. Following methods/techniques are generally applied to gain the aforesaid advantages, viz.:

1. Enema
2. Hip Bath
3. Sun-Bath
4. Fasting
5. Massage
6. Fruit and Vegetable therapy
7. Hot Foot-bath
8. Steam-bath

Enema

Spread a sheet on floor and lie on a hard surface, ensuring that your body touches the floor except hips, which should remain slightly elevated. Use a utensil which should hang down from a wall. Clear the tube, nozzle and utensil and let out some drops of water from the nozzle so that no air remains trapped therein. It will rule out possibility of air-pocket which shouldn't spill over to intestines and stomach. Now insert the nozzle into the rectum to facilitate free entry of water. When it is felt that requisite quantity of tepid water has entered the intestines, close and remove the nozzle and wait until pressure and urgency to defecate. Visit the closet when you feel it is no more possible to hold on water in the intestines. You may head even rumbling or gurgling sound of water in the stomach. Initially it may take some longer time to create urgency / desire for defecating but, when your intestines get used to enema water, such an urgency can surface earlier, with passage of time. To begin with, first of all water will gush out followed by stools of pasty or loose consistency. When you have emptied your bowels, give some rest to your body. In some cases one may have to visit the closet more than once which is quite natural and need not cause and upset or worry.

Persons, suffering from habitual constipation, may add ½ to 1 tsp of castor oil to water but no salt should be used. Enema must not be taken daily, but may be taken after 7-10 days, as daily enema use will make the intestines dependent thereof and one won't be able to pass stools without taking an enema. Those who are suffering from diarrhoea or dysentery must not take enema. Enema facilitates smooth passage of stools, doesn't let hard stools form, removes even chronic constipation, improves peristaltic action of bowels (intestines, rectum and anus). Enema must not be followed by fasting but one can take only light diet and some seasonal fruits and salads in moderate quantity. Avoid and resist the temptation of fried foods, fats, species, condiment, meat, fish or alcohol. Take only bland and easily digestible diet.

Sun-bath

Had there been no sun, there wouldn't have been any growth of vegetation, water wouldn't have flown down from the snow clad mountains, seasonal changes would have become a daydream. Infact sun protects, nurtures, develops, feeds, controls our various activities. Sunrise heralds advent of day and sunset indicates impending arrival of night. Sun-bath is a natural source of vitamin-D. It induces perspiration, thereby helping the toxins to excrete from our body, through skin pores. It also imparts much needed energy to our body. In a word, life wouldn't have been possible without sun.

Sun-bath is possible during winter days when natural heat is required by the body to sustain itself. In some rural areas people keep tepid water (stored in a bucket or some other utensil) under sun for 1-2 hours and then bathe naked / semi-naked in the sun. It has multifold advantages—Sun rays fortify medicinal properties of water, keep it lukewarm, solar energy (which consists of seven colours) reaches even minutest parts of our body and there is no fear of exposure. If whole body is massaged under direct sunlight / rays, oil will reach easily within our body, providing it a renewed energy and vigour. Further, all the skin pores will open and sweat glands get energised, sweating process will be activated so as to excrete toxins through skin pores.

Sun-bath has inherent therapeutic values, but in the west it is used as a cosmetic device only. In more sensitive persons sun-bath is not advised due to chance of exposure to cold, nor should they massage or take bath in the open. However, such persons should fully wrap up their bodies with a blanket if, at all, they are keen to have a sun-bath.

Fasting

It is a gateway to bliss and health. It not only purifies the body, it also purifies the man. In a way, it tones up, fortifies, purifies and sublimates body and mind. It takes away animal insights and inculcates higher values and laudable habits. To say that fasting is simply a way to starve the body is merely an attempt to under estimate it. Its importance lies in the fact that most, if not all, of the holy books laid stress on fasting and rightly iddised it as a gateway to heaven. Fast should never be implied to mean that it is simply a way to abstain from food rather to set in order all imprudent use of foods, besides removing acidity, gas, and flatulence. It corrects and tones up entire digestive system. In fasting, balance in body juices is moderated, improved, various mechanisms that produce blood, bones and flesh are totally corrected/overhauled, and cleansed, chemical balances brought under normal functioning. It also is a great purger of toxic elements, a great cleanser of filth, normalises and restorer of health, renders body agile and light. Moreover, our tired and overtaxed body and organs do get a well deserved rest. During the first two or three days, there may be felt some uneasiness, but regular practice will take away such element(s). It is said that -

"Whosoever fasts is blessed in every way as he draws the benefit of great medicines. All the diseases are cured and he becomes strong and virile".

Who Should not Fast

Following categories of persons should abstain from fasting process.

1. Pregnant and confined mothers before, during and after delivery and, more particularly, who are anaemic, emaciated,

and run-down and can't afford well balanced and nutritious food.

2. Mothers who are breast - feeding their infants.
3. Persons suffering from T.B., epilepsy, ulcers, labourers doing arduous manual work.
4. Persons during the course of actual travelling.
5. Old persons who are bed-ridden, unable to move, have stiff and immobile organs and eat far less than their actual requirement—in a way, the under and malnourished ones.
6. Weak, emaciated and starved children who are in their growth stage and also ladies belonging to that category.
7. Those who utilise fasting as a ploy for overeating and who indulge in dietary indiscretions.
8. Persons suffering from low blood pressure and low sugar levels in their blood.

Who should take to fasting

Persons whose condition and health state are reverse to the above persons can keep fasts. Following persons should take to fasting either completely, for the whole week, on all alternate days or, at least once a week or fortnight, depending upon necessity and urgency.

1. Persons who often overeat are gluttons.
2. Whose bowels are either impacted or often get loose motions.
3. Who suffer from dysentery, diarrhoea, colic, locking up of gas, rigidity of joints and other limbs.
4. Diabetics whose blood sugar level is generally high.
5. Habitual drunkards of alcoholic drinks, smokers, fast food eaters, obese and sedentary persons who eat too much but shun physical activity.
6. Children who are easy-going, relish foods prepared outside their homes.

What to do during Fasting

1. Mix a tsp each of lemon juice and honey in 150 ml water (cold or lukewarm) early in the morning and drink it. It will provide energy to the body. The same preparation may be repeated in the afternoon or some non-irritant liquid instead.
2. Do not remain stuck to chair or bed but attend to your daily chores, including physical activity.
3. Except when medically advised/necessitated, no medicine should be taken during fating—not even well exhorted tonics. Let by your physician be your guide in this respect, as far as use of medicine is concerned.
4. Fasting does not protract divorce from diet or any ingestion of food. Even while on fasts, you are allowed to take permissible eatable / drinks.
5. During summer season never starve your body from water which is our life force. There is no harm in taking a glass of orange or lemon juice which will help to purge our toxic, facial and unwanted matters from the body but will also strengthen the body.
6. No toxic food should be taken during fasting.
7. Fasting must not be utilised as an occasion and excuse for consuming fat-enriched, alcoholic, spicy, meat-based preparations or any other eatable which you have been forbidden.
8. If one wishes, one can resort to partial fasting for a week, each day you exclude one or two of these items iz. salt, sugar, grains, fats, spices, certain fruit or / and vegetable milk products. This way your body will have an almost disease free menu, when certain excess and shortages would be fully balanced. But a complete fast, at least once a fortnight or. When you exclude one or more items, you will yourself come to realise what item harms or benefits you and such a discerned conclusion should serve you as a guideline, enabling you to draw a long lasting food regimen.

9. Avoid alcohol and tobacco, drug and toxins, at least during the course of fasting.
10. Due care must be given to health status, age, sex, weight, work schedule and its demands on your energy expense. If you ignore such and any other viable factors, you will only expose yourself to problems which may lead you in a position of 'No-Return'.
11. Not taking anything during fasting or else overeating are the two extremes which should never be allowed to surface. Stick to what suits or does not suit you, instead of harping on what others say or eulogise or what is written in the books. It is reiterated that others' experience may be your nightmare or vice versa. It is your own body, and no one7 else could take care of it as you can, as you only know what is good or bad for you. You can always take a cue or inspiration from other person's personal experience and opinions but such averments cannot, and must not, be generalised. So, try to tailor all methods, opinions and suggestions to your own needs, depending on your own limitations, and compulsions. In short, try to be your own master. Listen to what others say or preach, but never succumb to temptations, avoid indiscretions and imprudent conclusions.

Fast, if stretched beyond your sustainable capacity, can be more harmful than 'no-fasting' approach.

Food

To keep your body in good humour, food is the most important factor. Truly speaking, 'we are what we eat' or 'our food habits mould our mental faculties also'. You can live without water for a few hours, without air for some moments and without food also you can survive, but merely survive. When body is not nurtured and nourished with suitable foods, our body gives in, giving way to many health problems. If body is not in a healthy state, mind also has to bear the brunt thereof, because a healthy mind lives in a healthy body. A lot has been written and spoken about food, proper food, food fads, fast foods, prohibited and acceptable and suitable foods. But, the fact remains that all foods do not and cannot suit all human beings as food allergies and reactions have a lengthy list of disorders. Naturopathy believes that most of our disorders stem from our wrong food habits and, vegetable and non-vegetable diets, are both the culprits in this respect.

Following points on food intake may be of help to the readers. (with particular reference to fasting under naturopahtic norms).

1. Take foods that suit you and, that too, at a particular time. If you have skipped a meal, there is no harm but overating or making up for the diet that you have missed is neither wise nor advisable.
2. Avoid all diets which abound in or contribute to formation of toxins, because once the body is ridden with poisonous elements, your entire energy would be expanded in getting rid of them.
3. Avoid white sugar but the same may be substituted with jaggery and sugar-cane juice.
4. Water of tender coconut will help to mollify acidity, restore normally to impacted bowels.
5. Milk curd, cheese and whey also help the body to purge out toxins from the body and also serve as mild and gentle laxatives.
6. Milk, curd, cheese and whey also help the body to purge out toxins from the body and also serve as mild and gentle laxatives.
7. Any food taken should not retard and impede the process of elimination which includes excretion of urine, faeces, phlegm, wind and perspiration.

Massage

Massage is a simple and effective method to attain and maintain ideal health. Therapeutic massage has been a well known method (that still exists in various cultures and civilizations dating back to thousands of years) profusely and frequently employed to promote general well-being. Self esteem, to boost immune and circulatory systems, to normalise blood pressure, remove extra fat content from the body, regulate respiration, improve digestion, muscle tone and skin tone. Different massage techniques have been successfully employed, developed and integrated into various therapies.

Key Principles

1. Massage can rejuvenate and invigorate body.
2. It can aid in relaxation of tired and aching muscles and painful and stiff joints.
3. Creates a sense of general well being and comfort.
4. Takes away tension from mind.
5. Lowers the amount of circulating stress hormones.
6. Promotes elimination of chemical wastes from the body, such as lactic acid which is said to lead to pain and stiffness in joints and muscles.
7. Opens up pores of the skin so as to help in inducing perspiration.
8. Improves mobility and flexibility.

Basic Techniques - Mainly our techniques are employed for massaging viz.:

(i) ***Stroking (or Effeurage):*** When hands glide smoothly and rhythmically over the skin, either in a circular or slow fanning motion or alternatively.

(ii) ***Kneading (or Petrissage):*** This action is like kneading a dough and hands are used alternatively to squeeze and release flesh rhythmically between the thumbs and fingers.

(iii) ***Friction:*** This method is employed for deep penetration, when even pressure is applied from the thumbs to a static point on the spine, or as small circles on the skin.

(iv) ***Hacking:*** Hacking is done with hands relaxed and working quickly over the skin. Here the side of the hands deliver alternate short, sharp taps on the body.

Vehicle used—Generally light vegetable oils or talcum powder is usually used as a vehicle for massage so that the hands glide over the skin. One may add essential oil to vegetable massage oil.

Precautions

- In case of any ailment, consult your doctor before embarking upon any non-conventional therapy.
- Do not massage during temperature rises, fractures, swellings, skin infections.
- Do not massage abdomen, legs and feet during first 3 months of pregnancy and, even after that, do not massage unless advised by a doctor.
- First get lumps and swellings checked by a doctor.
- Cancer patients may get massage, only if medically advised, from a trained practitioner only.
- Stop blending essential oil with vegetable oil, if any unusual symptom or discomfort is felt. Better consult a physician. Highly sensitive skins may even react to ordinary vegetable oils.

How to proceed

Some other person should do massage for another person because only another person can perform this job more efficiently and effectively. There must be a gap of 1-2 hours between massage and food intake. Always get body massaged on empty stomach, after attending to calls of nature, but without taking bath. Use a wooden plank or spread a thick blanket on the floor. Apply mustard / olive / coconut oil over skin and apply pressure equivalent to 5 pounds on tender organs and 5-10 pound pressure over hands, feet, abdomen and chest, 15-20 pound pressure over organs above waistline, like back, upper part. Actual pressure will depend on a person's physical condition. Fat accumulates generally around waist, abdomen, legs and arms, hence these body parts must be massaged more thoroughly. Some people advise inserting a few drops of mustard oil in ears, nostrils, navel, rectum but medical acceptance of such device still remain unconfirmed.

Our body has two extremities in the form of hands and feet as all the nerves end here. If palms of hands and soles of feet are thoroughly massaged, it will almost impart the benefits that are derived from Accupresure method. Message of palms and soles activates endocrine glands and all trigger points in the body, thus improving function of all the body organs.

Massage can be done from 15 to 60 minutes, depending on capacity of the patient and also the involvement of affected organs. After massage has been finished, relax for an hour or so, but do not drink / eat anything until you finish bath which may be had after an hour of the massage. Use some glycerine soap to remove residues of oily substance. Body massage should be done in the morning, 'before sunrise in the morning in summer season and after 2-3 hours of sunrise in winter season. Use lukewarm water for bathing purposes in winter or tepid water in summer. During massage, body sweats profusely and it is advised by experts that sweat should be reabsorbed into the skin; hence not wiped. Sivanand advised that, in order to ensure quicker penetration and absorption of massage oil, it should be mixed with some amount of table salt and also that oil may be heated or lukewarmed before being massaged.

Hydrotherapy

Hydrotherapy is an integral part of Naturopathy (other facets having been described earlier) and cold bath, hot bath, steam bath, sitz bath, alternate hot and cold baths, whirlpool bath, compresses, Turkish bath, steam room baths or steam bath by sitting / standing in a cabinet, saunas and wraps are the major disciplines. This therapy is deemed to be a complete healing system by which an ailing body, overloaded with toxic and foreign matters, can be eradicated from the body through skin pores in the skin by sweat in which is induced by hot / swim baths. This therapy is recognised both the conventional and non-conventional practice. Moreover, it is not new to India, Roman and Chinese who had been using it in one form or the other.

There is much evidence to prove that water has excellent ability to alter body's flow which could be manipulated varying its temperature, suiting an individual's capacity and health status. Cold water circulates blood to internal organs to enable them to reform their individual functions. It reduces blood pressure, increases blood flow to skin, dilates blood vessels, thus easing stiffness. It sends more nutrients and oxygen to the tissues, thus repairing the damage caused by various disorders. it also boosts immune system and improves blood circulation.

Mineral baths and mud have been known to allay tension, reduce circulatory congestion caused by spasm of muscles' and also are know to be beneficial in rheumatoid arthritis, better mobility and life of body joints. Some experts use cold and hot water alternatively.

Methods employed—

1. Sitz baths
2. Whirlpool baths
3. Hot or warm water baths
4. Alternate hot and cold water baths
5. Sea-water treatments
6. Wraps
7. Compresses
8. Turkish baths, Steam Room and Steam Cabinets.
9. Saunas.

Sitz Baths

Place two bath-lubs side by side—filling one with cold water and the other with hot water. The patient should sit for 3 minutes in hot water and one minute in cold water, keeping feet in the opposite bath. This position should be alternated.

Whirlpool baths

Immerse the body for 15 minutes in the pressurised bubbles and the body should be massaged.

Hot or warm water baths

Soak the body in hot water for 20-30 minutes, keeping temperature at 100°F or 38°C. If necessary oils, herbs and minerals can be added to warm bath. To derive better and quicker results, finely blended oatmeals / bran (possibly couched in a muslin bag) to soothe skin, and minds, and extracts (such as Dead Sea salts) to nourish the skin or Epsom salts to relieve the swollen joints.

Hot Foot Bath

Hot water should be used in winter and tepid water (if it is not too hot or cold) water in summer. Take a bucket wherein both feet can be immersed easily, and fill it to 3/4th capacity with suitable water adding, (if necessary), a teaspoonful of table salt. Now immerse both feet in the water, frequently massaging feet and legs in water itself. Keep the feet for about 20-30 minutes, and remove your feet from the water when it turns cold. (In winter cover your body with a blanket so as to avoid exposure). If you have added salt to water, then pour hot water over your legs and feet after removing the same from water. Thereafter, wipe with a dry towel. After wiping take care that feet and legs are not exposed to cold winds.

Alternate cold and hot baths

Alternate hot and cold water therapies are credited with the benefits or stimulating hormonal system, reduce circulation related congestion (caused by muscle spasm) and relieving inflammation.

Sea Water Treatments

Sea-Water is believed to possess healing properties while minerals inherent in seaweed are believed to induce sweating, tone and cleanse the skin. Seaside wraps, or sea water baths or sea-water itself, are also include in this system.

Wraps

In this process a cold flannel cloth-sheet is wrapped around the body and cold / hot packs are wrapped in towels for being placed on top. Then the patient is covered in a warm blanket and left for about 30 minutes. This process is employed to treat long-term fatigue, aid in circulation and to stimulate the immune system of patient.

Compress

Soak the towels in cold / hot water, wring out, and then apply to affected parts of the body so as to increase blood flow, make the body sweat and ease stiffness of muscles through hot compresses. Cold compresses are employed to reduce inflammation and push up circulation of blood.

Turkish baths, (steam) cabinets and steam rooms

If a patient sits in a steam room for about 20 minutes or for an hour in a cabinet, his sweat will be induced, impurities eliminated and water relieved. This procedure is known as Turkish baths.

Saunas

Though saunas are identical to Turkish baths but they generate dry heat and not humid heat. For Sauna, hot and dry temperature is required (say 100^0F or 38^0C). It encourages sweating and helps the body to eliminate waste products and impurities. After every 5-10 minutes during the sauna and at the end of the sauna, a dip or plunge into pool or cold shower is advised.

Precautions about the said devices

- During 1st trimester of pregnancy avoid sitz baths or steam baths, and during the next 6 months of pregnancy do not have treatments which exceed duration of 10 minutes.
- Patients of high blood pressure, heart disease or angina must avoid steam baths, saunas and hot baths.
- If a patient is asthmatic, epileptic, has undergone an operation or has a history of thrombosis, he must avoid all types of steam treatments.
- If one has an open wound, no ingredients should be added to bath. Patient who are allergic to iodine must avoid seaweed.

- Always consult and act upon the advice and guidance of a Naturopathy / Hydrotherpaist before embarking upon any of the discipline stated above.

Obese persons should weigh on a weighting scale daily, and thereafter every week to know that benefits have accrued and also what still needs to be done. One should aim to lose about one kg of body weight after a week and weight loss must be steady and gradual and never sudden and abrupt. Certain health clubs claim to shed enormous amount of weight within a week and often employ harmful techniques and strict dietary regiment to achieve their target which is not only undesirable but a health hazard also. Do not be misled by tall claims made by such weight reducing centres which have a covetous eye over your money. They are not concerned how much health and well-being you will have to sacrifice.

It is simply a matter of suitability as to which of the weight reducing devices and techniques could match with your physical competence; hence use your judgement in this regard but do not be missed by persuasion, publicity, big claims. If you wish, you may try your hand at western herbalists, Chinese herbalism, Auricular Acupuncture, Hypnotherapy, Homoeopathy, ayurveda, Tibetan Medicine-to mention a few only.

33

Bladder Infections

Bladder infections are caused by microorganisms that colonize the bladder in susceptible patients. Bladder infections may have no apparent symptoms even though bacteria can be cultured from the urine. Symptoms may also occur with no apparent infection.

Symptoms

The most common symptoms are urgent desire to urinate, frequent urination, bladder pain, low back pain, and burning pain before, during or after urination. Bladder infections occur most commonly in women following sexual intercourse, especially with a new partner. Bladder infections can also occur after waiting too long without urinating or going too long without drinking liquids. Catheterization is a common source of bladder infections in hospitals and nursing homes. Bladder infections often come on with sudden severity, but can progress gradually.

Complications

There is risk of bladder infections ascending up the ureter to cause acute pyelonephritis, a serious infection of the kidneys. Pain along the sides of the mid-back along with urinary frequency, urgency, and pain is indicative of a kidney infection and requires immediate treatment.

Finding the Homeopathic Medicine

— The most common medicines for bladder infections are Cantharis and Staphysagiria.

- Think of Apis if the pain is mostly stinging and burning, there is any swelling, the last drops feel scalding, and the urine will not come out easily.
- Give Cantharis if blood in the urine is prominent or the pain is excruciating. Cantharis has the most extreme bladder symptoms.
- If the major symptom is frequent, intense urging with very severe pain, give Mercurius corrosivus.
- Sarsaparilla is a very common medicine for women's bladder infections.
- If the major symptom is burning in the urethra at the close of urination, give Sarsaparilla. If it doesn't work, look at Staphysagria or Cantharis.
- If the bladder infection comes on after sex, consider Staphysagria first.

Self Care and Home Remedies

- Drink as much water as possible.
- Urinate whenever you have the urge.
- Avoid horseback riding or other activities that put pressure on the urethra and bladder.
- Take bladder herbs such as Oregon grape, Buschu, Pipsissewa, and Uva ursi every two hours until symptoms improve. The dosage will depend on whether it is a tea, capsule, or tincture.
- If citrus fruits aggravate your bladder, avoid them.
- Prevention suggestions include drinking liquids frequently and urinating as soon as possible after you feel the urge and after sex.

34

General Info About Hair Loss

Hair specialist (examining person's head). "Well, I am sorry, Mr. Rao, but your baldness has gone too far. I am afraid the only cure is a transplant. "Don't be daft man, I'd look bloody stupid with a kidney on my head."

Hair loss is one of the common problems among all of us. All hairs are shed at the end of their growth cycle, so some degree of hair loss is normal. If you have excessive hair loss, it makes sense to first understand the possible causes. There are many possible causes of hair loss, however most hair loss is normal, and part of each person's genetic program.

The most common type of hair loss is related to both genetic and hormonal make up, and is called androgen-dependent hair loss. About 50% of children with a balding parent of either sex will themselves become bald over a period of time.

Commonly used name for this type of hair loss is male or female pattern baldness:-

Male pattern baldness: Is characterized by a receding hairline, and moderate to extensive loss of hair, especially on the crown area.

Female pattern baldness: causes an overall thinning of hair on the head, and a moderate loss of hair on the crown or at the hairline.

What are the causes of Hair Loss ?

One of the primary cause of hair loss is a high amount of the male hormone, dihydrotestosterone (DHT) within the hair follicle. DHT is produced from testosterone in the prostate, various adrenal glands, and the scalp. After a period of time, an over abundance of DHT causes the hair follicle to degrade and shortens the active phase of the hair.

Another factor that has been linked to hair loss is the amount of sebum in the scalp. Sebum contains a high amount of DHT, and clogs pores in the scalp, both of which cause the malnutrition of the hair root. The amount of sebum in balding hair is related to the amount of oil in the hair. Meanwhile most doctors agree that frequent shampooing is advised in hair loss cases with oily scalps.

The most important cause of hair loss is inadequate nutrition. Even a partial lack of almost any nutrient may cause hair to fall. But hair grows normally after a liberal intake of these vitamins. A high protein and iron rich diet is recommended for hair loss. An adequate intake of raw vegetables, fresh fruits, salads, green leafy vegetables should be included in the diet on a regular basis.

Another important cause of falling hair is stress, such as worry, anxiety and sudden shock. Stress leads to a severe tension in the skin of the scalp. This adversely affects the supply of essential nutrition required for the healthy growth of hair.

General debility, caused by severe or long standing illnesses like typhoid, syphilis, chronic cold, influenza and anaemia, also gives rise to hair disorders. It makes the roots of the hair weak, resulting in falling of hair. An unclean condition of the scalp can also cause loss of hair. This weakens the hair roots by blocking the pores with the collected dirt. Heredity is another predisposing factor which may cause hair to fall.

How can Hair Loss be treated ?

The healthy condition of the hair depends, to a very large extent, on the intake of sufficient amounts of essential nutrients in the daily diet. Hair is made of keratin, a protein, which also makes up the nails and the outer layer of our skin.

A well Balanced Diet

Women require 60 grams, men 80 to 90 grams, adolescent boys and girls 80 to 100 grams of protein. It is supplied by milk, buttermilk, yogurt, soyabean, eggs, cheese, meat and fish. A deficiency of some of the B vitamins, of iron, copper and iodine may cause hair disorders like falling of hair and premature greying of hair.

Persons with a tendency to lose their hair should thus take a well balanced diet. An adequate quantity of vegetables seeds, nuts, green leafy vegetables, fresh fruits, egg and milk should be included in their diet regularly.

Surgical Hair Restoration

There are many surgical procedures which will help to restore the hair from falling. Surgical restoration is the only permanent solution to baldness. It involves a series of operations that extract plugs of scalp from the sides and back of your head, where hair grows densely, and implant them on top and in front, where you are going bald.

Scalp Reduction

Scalp reduction is performed on patients with well-defined bald spots in the crown area of the scalp. It is sometimes done in conjunction with hair transplantaion to reduce the size of the bald scalp, especially in patients who do not have enough donor hair to cover the bald areas.

Tissue Expansion

Silicon bags are inserted beneath an area of hairy scalp and gradually inflated with saline water over a six-week period. This causes the hair-bearing skin to stretch, thus increasing the amount of hair-bearing scalp. After removing the bags, expanded hair bearing skin is lifted and moved to an adjacent bald area where a similar sized patch of scalp has been excised.

35

General Info About Dandruff

Dandruff more scientifically called Seborrheic dermatitis is a disease that causes flaking of the skin. It usually affects the scalp. In adolescents and adults, it is commonly called "dandruff." In babies, it is known as "cradle cap."

Seborrheic dermatitis is a common skin disorder that can be easily treated. Dandruff appears as scaling on the scalp without redness. Seborrhea is oiliness of the skin, especially of the scalp and face, without redness or scaling. Patients with seborrhea may later get seborrheic dermatitis. Seborrheic dermatitis has both redness and scaling.

Know Your Skin

What are the causes of Dandruff ?

The basic underlying disorder is excessive oil production by the skin glands which in turn is acted upon by microorganisms, that might be a fungus, called Pityrosporum ovale. This organism is normally present in the skin in small numbers, but sometimes its numbers increase, resulting in the skin disease.

Dandruff appears as scaling on the scalp without redness. Seborrhea is oiliness of the skin, especially of the scalp and face, without redness or scaling. Patients with seborrhea may later get seborrheic dermatitis. Seborrheic dermatitis has both redness and scaling.

Dandruff causes embarrassment to the patient, in that it manifests clinically as intractable itching and deposition of greasy white scales which are dislocated from the scalp during the process of itching.

Dandruff (Seborrheic Dermatitis) affects the skin of the scalp, face, nose, eyebrows, behind the ears, external ear. Stress, fatigue, extreme weather, oily skin, infrequent shampooing, skin disorders such as dandruff and use of lotions that contain alcohol may increase the risk of seborrheic dermatitis. Neurologic conditions such as Parkinson's disease, head injury and stroke are also associated with seborrheic dermatitis.

How do we prevent Dandruff ?

There is no way to prevent or cure seborrheic dermatitis. However, it can be effectively treated. The tendency to develop this disorder appears to be inherited. The severity can be lessened by :

- Lessening stress.
- Avoid exposure to extreme weather.
- Use an oil balance formula for an oily skin.

How can Dandruff be treated?

The treatment of seborrheic dermatitis depends on its location on the body. Treatment also depends on the person's age.

This skin disorder is treatable but may recur. Gentle shampooing with a mild shampoo is helpful for infants with cradle cap. A low strength corticosteroid cream or lotion may also be applied to the affected areas of skin. Adult patients may need to use a medicated shampoo and a stronger corticosteroid preparation. Shampoo the hair vigorously and frequently. Loosen scales with the fingers, scrub for at least 5 minutes and rinse thouroughly.

Nonprescription shampoos containing tar, zinc pyrithione, selenium sulfide, sulfur and/or salicylic acid may be recommended by a dermatologist or a prescription shampoo may be given. However, patients should follow their dermatologist's advice, excessive use of stronger preparations can cause side effects.

More Valuable information about Dandruff...

Dandruff can appear on any part of the skin as patches of varying size. It manifests as white and yellow oily flakes associated with itching. Itching is usually harmless unless there is second degree infection associated. It may cause redness in the area affected with dandruff. Hair loss may also be associated with this disease.

Frequently asked questions about Dandruff...

a. Which specialist should I see if I have dandruff?

You should see a Dermatologist (skin specialist) and get their opinion.

b. Can people who have dandruff use a conditioner?

Yes, people who have dandruff can use a conditioner to keep up the condition of their hair. A conditioner does not stop the effect of an anti-dandruff shampoo on the scalp.

c. Is it true that the more lather produced when shampooing the more effective the shampoo is and the cleaner the hair?

No, the amount of lather produced has nothing to do with the effectiveness of a shampoo lathering agents are generally added to shampoos because people believe that more lather means cleaner hair and it tells the user where and when to rinse.

d. Is it true that the more shampoo you use the cleaner the hair will be?

No, a small amount of shampoo slightly larger than the size of a small coin and slightly diluted is usually sufficient for all hair at shoulder length that is washed frequently. The amount of shampoo will vary according to the length of the hair and how frequently it is washed.

Seborrheic Dermatitis—Skin condition characterized by greasy or dry, white scales. Dandruff and cradle cap are both forms of seborrheic dermatitis. Not contagious.

Dermatitis - Inflammation of the skin

36

General Info About Acne / Pimples

Acne known as pimples is a common disorder developed in teenagers and at times in young adults due to the inflammation of skin, as superficial skin eruption caused by the blockage of skin pores.

Usually acne appears on the face but can extend to neck, chest and back also.

Know Your Skin

What are the causes of Acne?

During adolescence, there is a sudden spurt in the secretion of sex hormones that cause increased formation of oils (sebum) from the sebaceous glands of the skin.

Sebaceous glands are secretory glands that open into hair follicles and skin pores. There is accumulation of oily secretions from the sebaceous glands due to blockage of the external pores in the skin. Consequently, the oils and dead skin cells are trapped, and form small "plugs" known as "comedones" within the hair follicles of the skin. Bacteria act on these plugs aggrevating the infection and causes the inflammation of the skin eruptions.

The plug causes the hair follicle to bulge causing white heads and if the top of the plug is darkened, it becomes blackheads. If the plug causes the wall of the follicle to rupture, the oil, dead skin cells, and bacteria found normally on the surface of the skin can enter the skin and form small infected areas called pustules also known as pimples or "zits".

Family history of acne can also contribute to the development of acne.

Other hormonal changes, can occur with menstrual periods, pregnancy, use of birth control pills, or stress and can aggravate acne.

What are the symptoms of Acne?

- Acne appears as rash on the face or neck. This rash can become a red and painful pustule.
- Presence of white heads and black heads can also lead to inflammation. Inflammation can be formed around the skin lesions.

How can we diagnose Acne?

Diagnosis is based on the appearance of the skin. Normally no tests are required.

How can Acne be treated?

Prevention—Treatment is designed to prevent formation of new lesions and aid the healing of the old lesions.

Medicines—that dry up the oil or promote skin peeling is applied on the affected part of skin. Antibiotics are applied if the acne is infected.

Surgical intervention—If the acne does not heal after a few days and produces cysts surgical intervention including professional (chemical) skin peeling, removal of eruptions, scars and removal or drainage of cysts is done.

Common facts about Acne

- Acne appears as white or red bumps and are painful to touch.
- Whiteheads are formed due to trapped oil and debris within the hair follicles of the skin.
- If whiteheads are formed in the deeper layers, a soft, fluctuant mass called a cyst appears.

- Blackheads are open and dark in color. This is due to melanin pigment and not dirt.
- The plugged wall of the follicle ruptures on to the skin surface, and can get infected by bacteria and form pimples or "zits".
- Small red bumps are called papules. Larger red bumps are called nodules.
- A pustule is a whitish yellow squeezable spot due to the accumulation of pus inside. After the lesions heal, they leave behind scars that form permanent marks on the skin.

Home remedy for prevention of pimples

- The tendency to develop acne is inherited. Although acne cannot be prevented, careful cleanliness can help to lessen the effects.
- Clean the skin gently but thoroughly with soap and water to remove dirt or make-up.
- Use a clean cloth to dry the face every day to prevent bacterial re-infection.
- Use steam or warm, moist compresses to open up clogged pores.
- Use topical astringents to remove excess oil.
- Don't squeeze, scratch, pick, or rub lesions. These activities can increase skin damage.
- Wash your hands before and after caring for skin lesions to reduce the chance of infection.
- Identify and avoid anything that aggrevates acne. This may include oily foods, lotions, make-up, and so on. Avoid greasy cosmetics or creams, which can aggrevate acne.
- Stress can add to the acne problem.

Frequently asked questions about Acne Pimples...

- Is it painful and contagious?

Acne can become painful but it is not contagious.

- Will it leave scars?

Acne can leave scars if they are squeezed or pricked.

- Are only teenagers affected by pimples?

No. Acne can be developed in any age though teenagers get it more frequently.

Sebaceous glands*—Secretory glands of skin that open into hair follicles and skin pores and are widely distributed on the body.*

Sebum*—Oily secretions of the sebaceous glands.*